The
Solution

The Solution

6 Winning Ways to Permanent Weight Loss

Developed at the University of California, San Francisco School of Medicine

Laurel Mellin, M.A., R.D.

ReganBooks

An Imprint of HarperPerennial

A Division of HarperCollins*Publishers*

A hardcover edition of this book was published in 1997 by ReganBooks, an imprint of HarperCollins Publishers.

THE SOLUTION. Copyright © 1997 by Laurel Mellin. All rights reserved. Printed in the United States of America. No part of this book may be used or reproduced in any manner whatsoever without written permission except in the case of brief quotations embodied in critical articles and reviews. For information address HarperCollins Publishers, Inc., 10 East 53rd Street, New York, NY 10022.

HarperCollins books may be purchased for educational, business, or sales promotional use. For information please write: Special Markets Department, HarperCollins Publishers, Inc., 10 East 53rd Street, New York, NY 10022.

First HarperPerennial edition published 1998.

Designed by Joseph Rutt

The Library of Congress has catalogued the hardcover edition as follows:

Mellin, Laurel.
    The solution : 6 winning ways to permanent weight loss / Laurel
Mellin. — 1st ed.
       p.   cm.
    Includes bibliographical references and index.
    ISBN 0-06-039186-3
    1. Weight loss. I. Title.
RM222.2.M4514 1997
613.2'5—dc21   96-50876

ISBN 0-06-098724-3 (pbk.)

02 ❖/RRD 20 19

To my parents, Rosabelle and Jack McClure,
my children, Haley, Joe, John and Riley,
my brother, Steve, and my "sister" Marguerite.
For their loyalty, their wisdom, and their love.

Contents

Part 4: A Clear and Simple Method

Acknowledgments

When I attended U.C. Berkeley in the late 1960's, a time of over-whelming chaos and social change, most of us thought the "system," the world our parents had passed on to us, didn't work. Now, reflecting on how *The Solution* has developed over nearly two decades, I find that the system, to my surprise, has worked decidedly better than we ever thought it would. This book—and the method on which it is based—is the result of a remarkable inter-mingling of the wisdom of many talented people and the support of a host of generous institutions.

Charles E. Irwin, Jr., M.D., Director, Division of Adolescent Medicine at the University of California, San Francisco School of Medicine (UCSF), not only hired me into a faculty position in the Department of Pediatrics in 1978, but allowed me to follow my interest in adolescent obesity. Through the awareness I developed in his division, I began to look at obesity not as a diet and exercise issue, but as simply another expression of the interaction of the mind, body and lifestyle.

Jonathan E. Rodnick, M.D., Chair, Department of Family and Community Medicine at UCSF, and earlier, Donald Fink, M.D., provided sanction and leeway for me to pursue my passion for understanding the mystery of weight problems. Marion Nestle, Ph.D., M.P.H., then Dean of UCSF's School of Medicine, and now Chair, Nutrition and Related Fields at New York University, saw something important in this work, and gave key support for continuing it during the leanest of years.

People Whose Ideas Guided the Way . . .

Jim Billings, Ph.D., whom I first knew in his role in the Preventive Medicine Research Institute and who became a cherished friend, generously shared with me his considerable insight into the interweaving of spirituality and health. His views have infused the entire book with greater depth and compassion. Carl Greenberg, M.S., of the University of Washington, Spokane, guided me in understanding family systems theory, and Jane Rachel Kaplan, Ph.D., author and eating disorder specialist in Albany, California, consulted on the developmental theories on which much of the method is based. John Gray, Ph.D., enhanced this work in many important ways, including impressing me with the importance of making requests of others and, in a larger sense, giving credence to the formidable power of seemingly simple ideas. Dean Ornish, M.D., and his ground-breaking program in heart disease reversal helped me understand the mind-body connection.

My agent, Robert Tabian, guided me—patiently and wisely—in creating my proposal and since then has been a constant source of support. Publisher Judith Regan not only understood and valued the method immediately, but developed a passionate commitment to bringing these ideas to every person who has ever struggled with a weight or eating issue.

Those Who Moved the Method Along Through Science . . .

Although *The Music Man*'s Professor Harold Hill used the "think method" with success, in developing this work we were fortunate to be able to build a theoretical framework based on research. For the research on the method and related work, I am most grateful to John Foreyt, Ph.D., and Ken Goodrick, Ph.D., of Baylor Medical College; Mary S. Croughan-Minihane, Ph.D., Larry L. Dickey, M.D., Lee Ann Slinkard, M.S., and Diana Petitti, M.D., all currently or formerly of UCSF; Patricia Crawford, Ph.D., and Zack Sabry, Ph.D., of the University of California, Berkeley; Elizabeth Brannon, M.S., U.S. Department of Health and Human Services, Bureau of Maternal and Child Health; and George Schreiber, Ph.D., of Westat.

The research of others, most particularly of Kelly Brownell, Ph.D., of Yale University; William Dietz, M.D., Ph.D., of New England Medical Center; Leonard Epstein, Ph.D., of the State University of New York at Buffalo; and, of course, Hilde Bruch, M.D., Dorothy Bauman, Ph.D., and Salvador Minuchin, Ph.D., was important in grounding this method in science.

Some Contributed Knowledge and Theory . . .

Some very knowledgeable people helped shape technical aspects of the method or its application to the young: Susan Johnson, M.D., Carl Baum, M.D., Felix Conte, M.D., Dennis Styne, M.D., Tom Boyce, M.D., Lane Tanner, M.D., Ronald H. Goldschmidt, M.D., Marna Cohen, M.S.W., Velia Frost, M.S.W., Carleen Goodwin-Hanson, M.F.C.C., Margaret McKenzie, Ph.D., and George Saba, Ph.D.

I am particularly grateful to Doris Derelian, Ph.D., R.D., for teaching me the value of the well-disciplined use of education theory; Francis Rapoport, Ph.D., for renewing my interest in cognitive therapy and her many insights as she co-led early groups; Daria Halprin, M.S., and Jennifer Harrison of Tamalpa Institute for consulting on the use of the expressive arts in the method; David Sheppard Surrenda, Ph.D., for sharing with me his views on the role of meaningful pursuits in health; Sharon L. Condy, R.Ph., for contributions in pharmacy; and Diane Schuette, M.S., for her insights on spirituality and eating.

There Was Important Organizational Support . . .

Several organizations supported or contributed to this work during its development, including the American Cancer Society, the American Medical Association, the American Dietetic Association, the U.S. Department of Health and Human Services' Bureau of Maternal and Child Health, the Preventive Medicine Research Institute, the Dairy Council of California, the North American Association for the Study of Obesity, the American Society of Bariatric Physicians, the American Academy of Pediatrics, the Healthy Living Institute, and the Public Health Foundation. To each of these organizations I am indebted.

. . . and Many Generously Supported in Other Ways.

For reviewing segments of the manuscript, I am particularly grateful to Larry Dickey, M.D., an expert on preventive health; David Gray, M.D., a family physician and obesity specialist; Stephen Woods, Ph.D., a University of Washington obesity researcher; and Edward Oklan, M.D., Helen Brown, M.P.H., R.D., Deborah Waterhouse, M.P.H., R.D., Francis Berg, M.S., L.N., Janice Lebeuf, M.P.H., Lonnie Barbach, Ph.D., Barbara McCarty, R.D., and Claudia Parker Lutz, R.D., M.P.H. The body pride stance was adapted from the work of Suki Munsell, Ph.D., *Dynamic*

Walking. Martha Weston contributed illustrations, and Trevor Ferruggia provided computer graphics.

Jennifer Gates Hayes deserves special recognition for her great care and sensitive attention in editing the manuscript. Ann Luckiesh, who reviewed the entire work and offered many astute reflections on it, saw these ideas from an entirely different perspective, nudging me in directions that widened the book's appeal considerably. Virginia Conlan had many valuable editorial suggestions. Karen Schanche, Martha Lunney, Pat Cherry, Lisa Reyes, Meg Kennedy, Kelly Masters, Jim Jacobs, Connie Bertrand, Kela Hicks, Janis Eggleston, Marlene Miller, Alicia Orellana, Kathy Small, Karin Hexberg, Nancy Nadaner, Leslie Tharp, Lois Bowman, Maeve Neuman, Michael Riordan, Michael J. Bjornson, Joel Miller, Susan Nutter, Dorothy Niehaus, Ruth Moore, and Sandi Smith offered their ideas and encouragement. Mel Lefer's kind support of the project was a much-needed gift.

Bob Mellin, my first publisher, shared with me the dream of changing the world for the obese young, and currently administers the professional programs that conduct groups based on this method. Resa Cherin has given countless hours to program research and service. Others have contributed their time and talents in important ways, especially Sharon Nielsen, Gretchen Vannice, Corinna Kaarlela, Brad Wong, Elyse Resche, Betty Herm, Elizabeth Dito, Robert Werner, Ann Vinson, Christine Cartright and Norisa Berardi. Peter Marguglio shared with me his courage and his caring, both of which I needed to write this book.

Family and Friends . . .

I am very grateful to my family. My mother found herself raising a daughter with unfortunate drives, and she gave me love—first by accepting my choices and then by devoting endless hours to listening to me deal with the consequences of them. From my father, I caught a passion for *doing something* in the world. He taught me the value of cultivating an understanding of people, and how to relax in the midst of chaos and settle into seeing the beauty and humor of it all.

My children bring me much of the joy that sustains me. I am thankful to Haley for her trust and friendship, to Joe for his patience and heart, to John for his exuberance and affection and for my memories of Riley.

I am grateful to my brother, Steve, for his honesty and love, to Vivian, for her loyalty, and to Sarah, Lisa and Michael. The legacies of Rosabelle Driggs and Laura McClure have been sources of inspiration.

I have had the grace of friendships with very special people, particularly Marguerite Moriarty, who truly is a sister to me and has comforted and laughed with me more times than I thought was humanly possible. Emily Kearney has continually shown me how natural it can be to love rather than judge and, in recent years, has coordinated many of our obesity conferences. Other friendships have warmed my days, especially those of James Patrick, Stephanie and Jim Moriarty; Andrea, Daniel, Sarah and Sophie Sharp; Nancy Heaton; Deirdre Taylor; Jock Begg; Sylvia Hughes; and Kathy McHenry.

Most Important . . .

I am grateful to each and every provider, participant and supporter who, over the years, believed in this method and saw solving weight problems as an opportunity to soothe the soul, mend the body and heal the mind.

Part 1
The Six True Causes

*How can we solve our weight problem if
we don't know the whole truth about
what is causing it?*

The Truth About Weight

I have identified a solution to weight problems, a way to end the agony forever.

The solution is not a pill, a personal trainer, or a diet shake. Nor does it require mustering willpower or acquiring true grit. The true solution to a weight problem is to cure all its root causes so that it has *no foundation* on which to rest. Then the weight problem has no choice but to *fall away* of its own accord.

What are the root causes of our struggles with weight? Apart from genetics there are six. Two are familiar aspects of our lifestyle: diet and exercise. Yet they are just part of the truth about weight. The other four—which typically aren't touched by weight programs—are the powerful mind and body forces that drive overeating and inactivity.

Quieting these forces eludes nearly every dieter. It is so frustrating! We *know* what to eat and how much to exercise—it's just that it is so hard to *do* it!

What Is the Solution?

There are six causes of weight problems. Each cause has a cure. When all the causes are cured, the weight problem is solved.

As it turns out, these mind and body causes are neither vague nor permanent, but very clear and quite open to change. In fact, each of these causes has a corresponding cure which is so simple that even children can use it with ease.

When all the mind and body causes of weight problems are cured, something profound happens: the drives that fuel overeating and inactivity stop. In their place arises a new sense of balance in mind, body, and spirit. We stop *wanting* the food so much. We stop *desiring* those nights on the couch.

Then, with only the gentlest of attention to enhancing the health of our lifestyle, the body's natural drive to reach a weight within its genetic comfort zone takes over. We not only shed extra pounds, but our weight problem feels solved.

You can solve your weight problem.

The idea of a weight solution is far from new. Each of us knows someone who has resolved their weight problem: they have lost weight and kept if off, and those troublesome drives to overeat and be inactive have long since stopped.

If you listen carefully to many of these people who have permanently ended their weight problem, they describe using a variety of supports—counseling, therapy groups, spiritual guidance or even lessons from the lumps and bumps of life. Yet their pathways—those inner shifts essential to their weight solutions—are all identical. *They are the six cures.*

These people found their own road to a weight solution. Unfortunately, their pathway was long and rocky, and they stumbled onto their solution by chance. You have a better option. You can use this method to walk a direct and certain route to your weight solution and reach it—not by *chance* but by *choice*.

Even though you may never have imagined that you could lose weight and end your weight problem forever, it is now possible to make that hope a reality.

This method, crafted over nearly two decades, the recipient of professional acclaim, the subject of more than seventy national conferences and used in hospitals across America, is now available to you in the privacy of your home through the pages of this book.

It's an inside job.

The reality that you can solve your weight problem easily may sound too good to be true. Like most of us, you may think of losing weight as a lifelong battle that can never be won—a personal purgatory of counting fat grams and forcing yourself to get off the couch.

In reality, the opposite is true. Not only do you have the power to lose weight permanently but that power doesn't come from struggling to "shape up" your lifestyle or surround yourself with a life free of changes, demands and stresses. It arises from the balance you create within yourself.

Yet, the cultural myth is that apart from genetics, weight problems are very *external* matters. Have you ever listened to your co-worker, best friend or mate explain why he or she gained weight? Chances are that person views the weight gain as the result of something external:

"I started traveling and I put on weight. It was those restaurant meals."

"I had a baby and haven't kept my weight off since then."

"My job takes so much time. I can't exercise consistently."

"If your mother-in-law moved in with you, you'd put on weight, too."

"My parents always rewarded us with food and made us clean our plates."

Such reasons sound plausible and familiar, but they mask the real engines that power weight gain. These lie not in whether we eat restaurant meals or have a demanding job, but in our internal environment—the inner processes that determine whether we react to these events in ways that cause our bodies to lose weight or gain it. That's why external solutions to weight problems lead to disappointing and even destructive results:

- We force ourselves to go on a diet while our emotional drives to overeat are still operating at full force. Of course, we can deny our needs for only so long until we relent and eat the whole mound of ice cream, the entire bag of cookies or as much bread as we can lay our hands on.

- We join an expensive gym with every intention of working out daily and looking buff and lean in a matter of weeks. We expect all this even though our internal controls still need some sharpening. Inevitably, we start bypassing the gym on our way home from work, then we chastise ourselves for being "lazy" and soothe our resulting guilt by sinking into an evening of watching television and eating pizza.

- We drink diet shakes for breakfast and lunch to "control" our eating. Yet our inner controls are in short supply and soon our body hunger is on the rampage. After a few days of being "good" and eating "sensible" dinners, we launch into an intense bout of lavish overeating that surprises even us.

So the first step in your weight solution is to understand the true causes of your weight issue—which are largely internal. This truth is phenomenal news for it offers immediate relief! *You can stop dieting.* Instead you will feel free to focus your energy on the remarkably easy and tremendously powerful changes that will bring you authentic and lasting success. In other words, your weight solution can begin.

What are the *true* causes?

If restaurant meals, work deadlines or your mother-in-law moving in aren't the true causes of weight problems, what are? Here are the six causes:

Mind

1. **Weak Nurturing**—If we don't nurture ourselves emotionally, we'll turn to something that is a universal satisfier: food. It will numb us, comfort us and become our best friend, but unfortunately, it will not fulfill us.

2. **Ineffective Limits**—If we don't set limits to protect ourselves from the demands of the world, we experience more stress in our lives—stress that is calmed by eating. Moreover, without being able to set limits on our own behavior, we're vulnerable to adopting the inactive, corpulent lifestyle of the average American.

Body

3. **Body Shame**—If we have little pride in our body or ourselves, what reason is there to push back from the table or sweat at the gym? If we ourselves don't matter, why should our weight matter? We skip the visit to the gym and have seconds when we really aren't hungry.

4. **Poor Vitality**—It takes physical vitality for a walk around the neighborhood to be a pleasure, not a chore. Without it we'll opt for the couch or the computer. And the number on the scale? It will increase.

Lifestyle

5. **Unbalanced Eating**—Without the skill of eating for health but allowing ourselves enough food pleasure to ward off feelings of deprivation, we are vulnerable to the seesaw of dieting and binge eating.

The Six Causes and Six Cures

The Causes	The Cures
MIND	
1. Weak Nurturing	1. Strong Nurturing
2. Ineffective Limits	2. Effective Limits
BODY	
3. Body Shame	3. Body Pride
4. Poor Vitality	4. Good Health
LIFESTYLE	
5. Unbalanced Eating	5. Balanced Eating
6. Stalled Living	6. Mastery Living

6. **Stalled Living**—There is a clear formula for living that guarantees we'll feel depleted and turn to food to replenish ourselves. That lifestyle involves little exercise, few meaningful activities and scant time to restore our bodies and spirits.

Each of these causes is very subtle, but when they work together they have the power to *cause* a weight problem. Conversely, when they are all changed only slightly, they have the power to *resolve* it. Yet without *all* the causes cured, the weight problem hangs on relentlessly and can never be solved completely.

This is a tremendous relief to know. It wasn't that we failed when we tried to lose weight but that our treatment only addressed *some* of the causes. With the powerful mind and body causes left to operate within us, it was inevitable that in time we would regain all the weight we had lost and more. It wasn't willpower that we lacked, but a treatment based on the whole truth about weight!

How did these causes develop?

The causes of weight gain are not part of character, genes or personality. They are *skills* that we didn't acquire earlier in life because of circumstances that were often beyond our control.

In a sense, possessing these skills is our birthright. It is our parent's job to guide us in mastering the basic skills of taking care of our health and happiness. But often our parents fall short of doing so, even though they did the best they could.

As we come of age, it becomes our task to take the baton from them and finish the job they started. Yet doing so is not easy, for often we aren't even aware of our patterns—they are so familiar to us and buried so deeply. And where to go to learn these skills isn't always clear.

Why didn't we acquire more of these skills in the early years? Not because our parents didn't *love* us. Most parents want to give their children a good start in life, and their good intentions often result in our having straight teeth, a college education and good manners.

Little did our parents know that what we needed—far more than a chiseled smile, a college diploma and no elbows on the table—was to master the six cures. For these skills protect us by building the inner resilience or personal Teflon that shields us from most problems—and enables us to bounce back from the rest.

Even if our parents knew what we needed, they may not have been capable of giving it to us. For unless they too have mastered the six cures, they automatically develop a style of parenting that trains us in the *causes* of weight problems, not the *cures*.

Essentially it comes down to this: If they have mastered the six cures, they will be responsive to our needs, and by the age of about six years we will have learned to take care of our health and happiness. We will quite naturally honor and express our own separate feelings and needs, set reasonable expectations for ourselves and have pride in our bodies and ourselves. From this will flow a reasonably healthy lifestyle. And chances are we will do well in life.

On the other hand, if parents haven't mastered these skills, they will be less responsive to our needs. They will be *permissive* or *depriving*—that is, they will give us too much or too little. Our parents will give us indulgence or neglect rather than nurturing, and harsh or easy limits rather than reasonable ones. Moreover, we won't master these six cures, and without our own personal Teflon to protect us, life won't go as well as it might.

Not only do we end up feeling alone, discouraged and numb, but we have other difficulties. We may gain weight if we seek comfort from food and solace from the couch. We may also have other symptoms of our lack of these skills, ranging from being the "good" child who achieves and "makes nice" to the "bad" child who acts out and has problems.

Perhaps we weren't even aware that we hadn't mastered the six cures until later in life when changes occurred: when our metabolism slowed; when the stresses and demands of life increased—whether through the birth of a child, taking on a new job or suffering the loss of a loved one. In these situations, we require more of these coping skills so that we are able to soothe and comfort ourselves rather than seek solace through the palate.

How are they cured?

Luckily, the six cures can be mastered at any age, for they are only skills, just like learning to ride a bike or swim in a pool. Also fortunately, these are *developmental* skills, the kind that once learned stay with us for life.

Why do these developmental skills have staying power? Because they are extraordinarily effective. Even the first time you use a cure, you'll notice an immediate benefit, which will encourage you to use it again. Soon you'll use the skills so often that they become totally unconscious and part of your natural functioning.

Just recall other developmental skills you've already mastered, such as walking. When you took your first wobbly step, it worked! That step moved you across the floor more quickly than crawling, so you took another and another until you were walking all the time. Moreover, you didn't even consider going back to crawling, because it didn't work as well. This is precisely what will happen as you master the six cures.

Let's pause for a moment. This means that the core of your weight solution is *not* to force yourself to eat carrots instead of cookies and pry yourself up off the couch to go for a run. Instead it is to enhance your skills in the six cures until they become so natural that they work internally to slowly melt away any extra pounds.

What a relief! You do not need to deprive yourself in order to lose weight. Your own inner strength and wisdom—gently fine-tuned by these cures—will solve your weight problem in ways that brute force or steely willpower never can. The result? The number on the scale will drop. And the experience won't be grindingly hard. The lost weight may even seem like an afterthought, a side effect of small but powerful adjustments within.

What's more, since the root causes of being overweight are embedded in the body, mind and soul, solving weight problems frequently triggers a broad spectrum of life changes beyond weight. In a somewhat miraculous turnabout, weight loss stops being a chore that deprives us of life's pleasures and starts being a rewarding and even fascinating opportunity to heal and strengthen the very foundation of the self.

Fortunately the method is universal.

"But will it work for me?" you might be asking. In a word, yes. Mastering the method will not overpower Mother Nature and genetics, but it will guide you to shed more easily any excess body weight—*no matter who you are or what your weight problem.*

It doesn't matter whether you are trying to lose the last five pounds, end a compulsive eating problem or take off more weight than you ever imagined you would carry. The same six cures apply, regardless.

Likewise, the labels society uses to separate people don't have any place in this method, because gender, race, ethnicity, religion or income are not at the deepest roots of weight problems.

Nor is personality. These same causes appear to push up the number on the scale regardless of the diverse spirits standing on it. Compare the factors other than genetics that add pounds to Ricki Lake vs. Oprah Winfrey, Rush Limbaugh vs. Jay Leno and Margaret Thatcher vs. Elizabeth Taylor. You will be likely to find the very same roots.

How can one simple method work for so many problems and such a diversity of people? Because these powerful cures have their basis in human nature. They are the most basic internal skills all humans need in order to protect, honor and empower themselves. As a result, in matters of weight, there is union among us.

On a personal note . . .

Part of my pleasure in sharing the method is that I know first-hand what it does and can anticipate the rewards it can bring you. As a teenager, I was saved from becoming seriously over-weight only by a combination of skinny genes and nutritional savvy. However, my emotional appetite for sweets was more than a little frightening, and I thought of it as a curse that I'd have for the rest of my life.

As a young faculty member at the university, however, I began to unearth the true causes of weight problems from the depths of the mind-body literature. It didn't take more than scratching the surface of my awareness to see these root causes in myself.

How often I had disregarded my feelings and needs and set harsh limits for myself. How frequently I had disparaged my body and paid little attention to my health. No wonder my life at times felt chaotic and empty and my thoughts turned to food far too often. Now I could see that my power was not in thinking about my next meal—what I "should" and "shouldn't" have—but in hon-oring my feelings and needs and being easier on myself.

I began to use the tools of the method in my own life. With some surprise, I watched my drive to overeat begin to wither, and my discomfort with my body size wane. More important, my day-to-day life was better, and a comforting sense of balance and presence visited me more often.

At that point I started what felt like a rebuilding process—taking better care of my health and eating prudently, exercising regularly out of self-love rather than because I "should." In the end, my weight stabilized at a level that was well within my genetic comfort zone and I felt . . . *cured.*

I also felt grateful. Because clearing away the last evidence of my weight problem, which had seemed like such a curse, ended up being a blessing. My weight was just what I needed: a symptom distressing enough to stimulate me to change in order to solve it. Not by coincidence, those inner changes ended up being precisely the ones I most needed to make in order to make my life better.

When my own weight issues resolved, I looked back over how much of my personal energy had been sidetracked by my weight. Far, far too much of it. There are millions of us who dieted just the way I did—over and over again without success. *Millions!* What a tremendous loss of time, energy, and more important, spirit.

In the past, we dieted and indulged and fretted and fumed because we didn't know a better way. Now we do. Given the power and simplicity of *The Diet-Free Solution,* none of us—including you—needs to suffer that agony any longer.

What Are the Six Cures?

The cures are not medical breakthroughs, exotic drugs or spiritual events. They are a cycle of three questions that you can ask yourself at any time of the day or night to return yourself to balance in mind, body or lifestyle. The answers to the questions will vary widely, but the questions remain the same regardless of your situation or circumstance.

Moreover, you do not need a stack of textbooks to answer the questions, for you will soon find that you possess all the answers. All you needed was these tools—the cures—to fully access the wisdom, strength and goodness that was within you all along.

In this chapter, I will escort you through the experiences of two people who have mastered the six cures of the method. You will see how each of them used these cures to solve their weight problem and reap some unexpected rewards along the way.

"I'm totally out of control with food, and I hate my body."

Stacy was a 30-year-old interior designer. She had a caring husband, Thomas, and a lovely 6-year-old daughter, Lisa. Stacy was used to overeating to soothe herself when she felt depressed, anxious or tired. But even as the food calmed her, overeating stirred frightening feelings of being out of control.

As Stacy's weight went up and her clothes got tighter, Thomas saw his wife's intense frustration and the shame she felt about the size of her body. Stacy felt completely helpless to do anything about it, and told Thomas repeatedly how scared she was of passing the "curse" of her eating and weight issue on to their daughter.

"I like ribs and steak more than lettuce and sprouts. Who doesn't?"

On the other hand, George wasn't bothered by his weight. At 48, he had a successful track record in the advertising industry, and he saw himself as happy and fortunate. He had a fine marriage to Barbara, a real estate agent, and good relationships with his sons Ben, age 13, and Josh, age 11. George thought of his large stomach as a simple matter of liking ribs and steaks more than lettuce and cucumbers.

Now let's examine each of the six cures and the ups and down that Stacy and George experienced as they mastered them.

Cure 1. Strong Nurturing

Effectiveness in getting your needs met.

3. Support   **1. Feelings**

2. Needs

Nurturing isn't *indulgence*. It's taking care of our own needs.

The first cure is Strong Nurturing. Nurturing is not just what parents do to babies but also the opposite. It is at the root of establishing autonomy from our parents so we are less dependent upon others to meet our basic emotional needs.

We can rely on ourselves because we have an inner voice that affirms us and attends to our needs. Oddly enough, needing others *less* enables us to open up to them *more* because we have less fear that they will reject us or that we will surrender to their will. What's more, we can finally stop worrying that if we open the door to our hearts even a crack, others will discover how negative and judgmental we are. This is because our inner lives become—more often than not—positive and accepting.

What happens if nurturing isn't our strong point? We are vulnerable to developing emotional or "stress" appetites. And among Americans the most common excessive appetite by far is for food—at least 50 percent of American adults admit to using food binges to cope with the stresses and strains of living.

Frankly, in the absence of more effective ways of soothing ourselves, overeating is a reasonable choice. Anyone who has ever finished off half a pizza or a pint of chocolate ice cream knows that eating is *very* soothing. And distracting. And gratifying.

It celebrates our highs and buffers our lows and removes us from the frightening intensity of being alive. Or perhaps eating is the only time we are intimately aware of life's bounty. The pleasures of the palate and the reassurance of feeling full may be how we feel alive, secure and loved.

"I'm so depressed. I want these cookies. I need these cookies. I'm going to have these cookies!"

"What do I need? Intimacy—but I rarely have it, so I stay up late at night watching television and having something good to eat."

"I don't want to feel this much. It's too intense. I need the food for a release."

When I first suggest to participants in Solution groups that they can soothe, comfort and pleasure themselves without overeating, they don't believe me. If they were truly nurturing themselves, they say, they'd never *stop* eating. Yet that is not our experience with those who master the method. Strong nurturing enables us to identify our true needs—which are masked as a desire to eat—and meet them. Eating is an important sense of pleasure, but not the centerpiece of life's comfort.

How do I feel?

The nurturing cycle involves being aware of feelings as they arise throughout the day. The answers to this question will open up new possibilities in your life because you have started your query by digging way down deep inside to your feelings.

The basic feelings you discover there are weather vanes that point to your inner state more accurately than thoughts. As a result, even the socially unacceptable feelings—anger, sadness, fear and guilt—are tremendously cherished because they clear away the inner turmoil and cut a direct path to identifying what you *really* need.

What do I need?

Our next challenge is to discover what we *need* that could best satisfy our feeling. For instance, food saves us from hunger, but it's a poor life raft for feelings of anger, sadness, fear, guilt and joy.

Often the need is simple: when we're tired we need sleep, and when we're bored we need an interesting activity. Other times our need is abstract. When we feel sad, we don't just need to talk with our partner. We need our partner to listen to us with respect and empathy—and without half their attention on the kids, the television or their work.

Unless we *know* what we need, we rarely get it. It's not only difficult to follow through and meet a need if we're not sure what it is, it's impossible to ask for support in meeting it!

The fact is that it's difficult at first to pinpoint our needs. Do we *really* need this or do we just *think* we need it? Is this something that is *reasonable* to need or a "greedy" indulgence? Fortunately, like all of the questions of the cures, the more often you approach yourself with respect and ask this question, the more rapidly your answers will become both accurate and clear.

Do I need support?

As competent adults we can meet many of our needs ourselves. Yet if we take the next step and ask for support from others, the rewards are far greater. In fact, last week in our group, two people approached me separately and said, "Do you know what makes the most difference for me?" I said, "No, what?" They gave the same reply: "Asking for support."

There are obvious reasons: it's nice to have our own way and it's helpful to receive support. However, requesting support has far more earth-shaking rewards in store for us, and they're ours *literally* for the asking. Each time we make a request of others, we are affirming our:

- *Right* to have needs

- *Responsibility* for taking control of getting our needs met

- *Capacity* to soothe ourselves if our request is denied

This opens the door to intimacy in two ways. First, others sense that we know how to take care of ourselves. Closeness with us will not result in a cascade of our needs gushing out—with the unstated expectation that the other person will rescue us by meeting them.

Second, we are not rigidly, perfectly and sadly independent but vulnerable enough to *need* someone. The success ethic implies that if we are only "good enough" we will merit love. In fact, the opposite is true. People love us not because we are *good*, but because of our vulnerability, our *humanness*. When we come off the pedestal of self-sufficiency by making a request, we show that humanness, which inspires others to love us more.

"He acts like everything is fine."

At first, George's view was that nurturing wasn't relevant. He had all the nurturing he needed: a loving wife and two great sons. Barbara saw it differently: "George comes home from work as tight as a drum and digs into his dinner like it was his last meal. He acts as if everything is fine when I know it isn't, except occasionally when he really blows his top and scares the kids—and me too."

"She would take emotional nosedives . . . "

Stacy rarely nurtured herself, and inevitably she would sink into emotional lows, complain to Thomas and seek solace in food—mainly cookies and candy bars. According to Stacy, her moods affected Thomas and her daughter, Lisa, too. Thomas felt frustrated that he couldn't help her, and Lisa cried more than usual, as if her mother's sadness was catching.

Cure 2. Effective Limits

The strength to follow through.

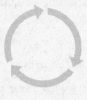

**3. Essential
Pain**

**1. Reasonable
Expectations**

2. Positive, Powerful Thoughts

Limits bring us safety and success.

The second cure, Effective Limits, is the cure that takes our raw feelings from the nurturing cycle and "grows them up." It bolsters our sense of power, personal fortitude and capability to produce success in our lives.

I've always considered my basic nature to be a little oversensitive, somewhat passive and bordering on wimpy. Yet what amazes me is how the limits cycle can make me strong—like an immediate source of "spinach."

When I'm feeling like Olive Oyl tied to the train tracks screaming "Help! Help!" the Popeye within me downs that spinach and comes to the rescue, bursting those ropes and rescuing the damsel. The only difference is that I don't have to always wait for Popeye to save me—*the limits cycle gives me the strength and power to save myself.*

Are my expectations reasonable?

The first part of the limits cycle is to set ourselves up for success by having reasonable expectations. This sounds like an easy call, but it isn't. If one is raised with expectations that are too high or too low—or a seesaw between the two—the middle ground, what is *reasonable*, is not at all familiar. Yet finding that midpoint of reasonable expectations is essential to success. Here's why:

If our expectations are too low . . .

If our expectations are too low, even if we follow through, we'll fall short of success. For instance, we may roll along in life not exercising but unconsciously expecting not to gain weight. The result is that we don't exercise and we gain weight, then feel somewhat confused about how that happened and a little disappointed in ourselves.

What's so fascinating is that often what seems like *low* expectations are actually *no* expectations. In a particular area—whether it is exercise, intimacy or savings—we have no clear expectations of ourselves at all. We have never looked deeply inside and said to ourselves, "Okay, I know what society expects, what my mother and father expect and what the doctor expects, but what in the world do I expect of myself?"

With easy or unclear expectations, inadvertently, we deny ourselves the first step in gaining control of our weight and our lives. We haven't put the ball into play so we can't possibly hit a home run and experience the success we desire.

If expectations are too high . . .

Contrary to the claw-yourself-to-the-top mentality that is pervasive in our culture, expecting too much of ourselves is as ineffective as having low or no expectations. What happens if our expectations are too high? We procrastinate, give up or harm ourselves in the process of meeting those elevated goals. In any of these cases, we rarely win the happiness and health we deserve.

Dieting is a prime example. We expect too much of ourselves, such as to subsist on veggies, fruits or paltry amounts of food all week—eating like a bird and losing the weight—but end up missing the joy of living because we are grouchy, weak and miserable. Instead, we may anticipate the pain of denying ourselves the satisfaction of food and stay entrenched in unhealthy eating patterns. In all these instances, those harsh expectations have been thick blockades that separate us from sucess.

Is my thinking positive and powerful?

We can be our own worst enemy or our own best friend. What this old truism refers to is the voice inside our head and whether the voice is negative and powerless or positive and powerful.

If those inner messages are negative and powerless, it won't matter a hoot if we are blessed with an adoring spouse, a bungalow in the South of France and a blank check at Bloomingdale's. Happiness will elude us because we are *living* with the enemy—ourselves.

And we can't afford to live with the enemy, because life is tough, and it's hard to cut up vegetables when we feel like a slice of pepperoni pizza dripping with melted cheese. It's not easy to rush home after work, throw off the suit, the tie, the heels or whatever, slip into running clothes and hit the gym rather than the sofa.

So the challenge, in order to follow through with our noble plans of eating right and exercising regularly, is to notice what that voice inside is saying and *make sure* that it's helpful!

We need to replace the negative thoughts with positive ones and make the powerless ones more powerful—much like a mental gardener: First we yank out the weeds of those judging, perfectionistic, helpless thoughts. Then we plant and nourish the positive, accepting and empowering ones. The result? Our garden flourishes quite nicely.

In the same way, we cut up the vegetables, go to the gym and watch our waistlines grow smaller and smaller.

What is the essential pain?

According to Scott Peck in *The Road Less Traveled*, life is difficult, and accepting rather than resisting that reality makes everything a little easier. The skill of facing the pain inherent in the situations life presents—from getting a flat tire to losing a loved one—is the most powerful part of the limits cycle. What I call "essential pain" is the unavoidable reality one must face in order to go forward. Facing that essential pain requires recognizing what that reality is and having the composure to experience the feelings that follow that realization—and staying with those feelings until they naturally fade. Often the essential pain is that we aren't perfect, we can't control everything, the past can't be changed or future disappointments could occur.

We usually avoid essential pain at all costs—and the costs are typically extraordinary, including not only weight issues but most struggles with excess. We fear that if we really felt our essential pain it would grab us, shake us and never let us go. In reality, if we are willing to feel our essential pain it does fade.

For instance, the essential pain of getting a flat tire—that we aren't in complete control—results in anger. The feeling of frustration rises and falls. If we can feel that feeling and let it wash over us, when it fades our sense of control and balance rushes in. The experience is truly remarkable.

That small skill is so empowering that when we practice it in Solution groups, the reaction of participants is always strong and always positive. The common response is, "I feel relieved. I feel strong. I feel great! Thank you!"

Too hard on himself at work and too easy on himself at home

George had a style of setting limits that was far too harsh at work and too easy at home. At work, he thought he could control everything and was unwilling to accept the essential pain that deadlines sometimes weren't met and people weren't perfect. At home it was a different story. George felt guilty about his long hours of work and the stress he brought home with him. He set few limits with Barbara and the boys, allowed them to overspend financially and set no limits on his eating, drinking or lack of exercise. None.

"Do it perfectly . . . or don't bother doing it at all."

Stacy expected far too much of herself. In her mind, there were two ways of doing something: perfectly or not at all. Her thoughts were so full of perfectionism that she had little emotional reserve left to face follow-through. She made valiant attempts at impossible goals, couldn't possibly meet them and, as a result, sank into a depression, which she cushioned by eating.

When I honor my body, I honor myself.

Body image and self-image are so thoroughly intertwined that a negative opinion of the body is a direct slam to the ego. In the absence of the third cure, Body Pride, self-esteem dwindles and

Cure 3. Body Pride

Honoring and accepting your body.

3. Honor and Accept　　　　**1. Avoid Weightism**

2. Use Words, Not Weight

takes with it any fledgling attempts to eat healthily and exercise well. When body pride wanes, the last ten pounds won't budge and larger amounts of weight are often held on to with a tenacity that is subconsciously fueled by rage or despair.

For some people, body pride seems like a mirage in the desert, something they can envision but never reach. The fact is that body pride—like pumping iron or baking a cake—is a skill that is well within their grasp.

Am I avoiding weightist thoughts?

Weightism is discrimination based on body weight and, of course, is no less despicable than racism or sexism. Unfortunately, it is ubiquitous.

The first part of the body pride cycle keeps the poison of prejudice at bay by *starting with ourselves*—that is, by tossing out our own weightist thoughts and substituting thoughts that are accepting and supportive.

For instance, we can switch the weightist thought "*You're too fat*" to the body pride statement "Your *body is OK regardless of its size.*" Or change the weightist thought "*People will notice I've gained weight*" to the body pride statement "*Other people's weightism is their problem, not mine.*"

Am I using words, not my weight, to express myself?

Often people can't stand their extra pounds and want nothing more than to shed them, like water off a roof. *But somehow it doesn't happen.* And the most common reason is that being overweight, on a subconscious level, helps them. Maintaining a larger body size speaks for them without their having to use words.

What we use our weight to say for us varies from person to person. To a spouse in a disappointing relationship it might say, "I don't want intimacy." Body size may be a silent message to a critical parent, "You can't control me," or to clients, "I am powerful." What we are saying doesn't matter. What does matter is that we find those words and say them, so that we don't have to use staying bigger than the size that is best for our health and happiness to do it for us.

When we find those meanings and express them with words, the extra body size is no longer needed, and we begin shedding pounds effortlessly. It's amazing! The weight comes off spontaneously, just the way we'd naturally discard a thick wool coat in a blazing hot room. Because the weight, like the coat, is no longer needed.

Am I honoring and accepting my body?

The last part of the body pride cycle is to honor and accept our bodies. On a very practical level, this means going to the beach, taking that job, or dressing like dynamite *now*, instead of waiting until some mythical time in the future when we are finally *perfect*. It's switching the inner voice to accept genetics and honor our bodies as they are right now, *imperfections and all.*

Honoring and accepting our bodies takes us by the hand and helps us step off the drive-for-perfection pedestal. We emerge from the cloud of self-hate and in an odd turnaround lose weight rather than gaining it. Why? Because from body acceptance flows self-acceptance. Equipped with more self-respect, we wince at the idea of overeating, cringe at the thought of spending evenings on the couch, wondering, "Why would I *do that* to myself?" In essence, the love of self heals.

***His days of athletic glory and sensuous marathons
were over.***

During the years that George was overeating, he didn't
pay much attention to his body from the neck down. Why
should he? He was less preoccupied with a romantic
interlude than before and the athletic glories of high
school football were long gone, so where was his motivation to be another Rocky and get in shape? Moreover, his
size had an advantage. In a subtle way, it made him feel
stronger and more powerful.

"I judge myself by my weight. I always have."

Stacy was completely open about her weightism: "I
judge people by their weight, the same way I judge myself."
Moreover, keeping on those extra pounds and complaining
to Thomas about her powerlessness over her weight was a
way of saying to him, "I need you. Help me." Finally, Stacy
had inherited her mother's rounded hips, and her rejection
of them added to her low sense of worth. Her sadness
about her imperfections sent her down the path to depression and overeating. She needed desperately to give her
body and herself the warm acceptance it would take for her
to look in the mirror and say, "Round hips? Yes, that's me!"

Cure 4. Good Health

Optimizing your physical vitality.

**3. Health
Care**

**1. Body
Awareness**

2. Self-Care

Give me a little vitality, I'll give you a thinner shape.

Any stumbling on the pathway to physical vitality can put out the welcome mat for weight gain.

The cause of our health malaise matters little. Anything from a throbbing headache to low fitness can put us over the edge. We don't make a salad for dinner, but instead call out for pizza. We think about taking a walk after dinner, but settle into an evening at the computer instead. As a result, the fourth cure is seizing Good Health, that is, all the physical vitality within our reach.

How does my body feel?

Just the way the car coughs a couple of times and drags a little before it needs a tune-up, so too does the body send out subtle messages that we're not well, which we must heed to optimize our health. The first part of the good health cycle is to check muscles, bones, organs and skin and listen attentively to any warning signs, so we can take early and effective action to guard our vitality.

Am I taking care of my body?

The second part of the good health cycle is to take care of ourselves, which is even more of a challenge for those of us with weight concerns. Even though the crux of this part of the cure is being your own health advocate, along with extra weight comes a greater need to *know*.

For instance, are there drugs or health problems that add to your weight, or medical conditions you thought wouldn't come for decades that have arrived far too early? If so, doing all you can to minimize their impact on your vitality is essential.

Is my health care effective?

When was the last time you had such excellent heath care that you knew you were as healthy as medical science would allow?

The truth is, most of us are ineffective health care consumers. We don't stick up for ourselves, we don't ask to be spoken to in plain English, we don't request that the doctor recommend alternative therapies—whether it be yoga for heart disease, support groups for breast cancer or drinking plenty of water for a slow digestive tract.

This part of the good health cycle involves boosting skills to ensure that our health care is as effective as we deserve it to be.

"My health is great. Really it is . . . "

When I asked George, "How is your health?" he responded with a resounding, "Great!" It was only after we talked further that I discovered that his eating and drinking left him lethargic in the evenings, with barely enough energy to watch television. In addition, nagging backaches made exercise painful, and although his doctor had given him back exercises that would help, he never did them.

"The doctor wouldn't listen to me . . . "

For such a young woman, Stacy had a surprising cluster of health problems that dragged her down. Her PMS was vicious for a week every month, yet her doctor had little interest in her symptoms, so Stacy just endured it. What's more, highly seasoned foods made her sick, yet she still ate pizza and garlic bread and lived with the miserable aftereffects on many evenings. Finally, she had lots of unanswered questions about weight loss pills. Did they work? Were they effective?

Getting science on your side . . .

You can eat almost any food—if the amounts are small enough—and still lose weight. However, dieting on candy bars or on one big dinner at night has its price: the discomfort of hunger, energy drains and fuzzy thinking, as well as a greater chance of gaining it all back.

When the chemistry of food and the biochemistry of the body are in synchrony, weight loss is far easier. That's just half the story, of course. Eating is also about pleasure, gratification, artistry, romance, community and celebration. The balanced eating cycle is a way of heeding the advice of nutrition science while accepting the imperfection of being wonderfully human, the side of us that eats with abandon.

Cure 5. Balanced Eating

Eating for health and pleasure.

3. Health and Pleasure

1. Regular Meals

2. Hunger

Am I eating regularly?

Eating at regular intervals throughout the day makes biochemical good sense. The starve-all-day, eat-all-night pattern overloads the liver, demands that it store food as fat and prompts more eating at night, the time when fat cells are most apt to grow larger.

Furthermore, eating regular meals means *not eating* for regular intervals, which can mean *not having to think* from moment to moment, "Shall I have something now? What will I have now?" Since just thinking about eating can trigger changes in insulin and the hormones that stimulate appetite, eating regularly cuts down on the false hunger that prompts us to eat when our bodies have had enough.

Am I eating only when I am hungry?

Eating when you are hungry and stopping when just satisfied, waiting ten minutes and noticing whether or not you are full, is the easiest way to keep our energy high while we gradually lose weight. You'll revel in the ease of it. No more counting servings, scrutinizing fat grams or fretting about portion size. Just as your ancestors did for eons, you will trust your body and yourself!

What's the catch? Your body's signals need to be fed a steady diet of . . . eating regularly, avoiding overeating and getting plenty of exercise to accurately reflect your need for food. But that won't be difficult, for as you progress in mastering the mind and body cures, you will live in a healthier way quite naturally.

Is my food both healthy and pleasurable?

Ripe strawberries, fresh bread and succulent chicken—there are so many healthful foods that bring pleasure and can be the cornerstones of your eating. The challenge is to eat as healthfully as possible but to eat enough of the more luscious foods to prevent any trace of a feeling of deprivation. In other words, we must know how to eat for both *health* and *pleasure*.

The Solution food list makes eating for health easy. It is based on a way of eating that is low in fat, moderate in sugar and protein, high in substances called phytochemicals that protect against disease and adequate in all the essential nutrients.

Moreover, this way of eating is completely nondepriving. Not only are there no forbidden foods—all depriving ourselves does is make us want them more—but you will not be *encouraged* to eat foods that are nutritional disasters.

Why? Because you are more important than your food and your weight. It is essential to a weight solution to honor yourself. Denying our need for an activity as primitive as eating conjures up feelings of rejection and distrust—a reminder of the worst moments of childhood. Those feelings alone are enough to trigger an appetite for the forbidden that knows no bounds!

"It's funny, but when I really think about it, do I really *need* that food? Not really."

"I usually overeat out of habit. It's natural to me. But when I ask myself if the essential pain of not overeating is too difficult for me, I usually answer no. Then I end up not eating the food after all."

Oddly enough, this stance toward food actually promotes losing weight because the dynamic around food begins to change. When you *always* honor your need for food, you don't *always* want the most luscious ones. After all, those foods don't serve your needs for vitality—and therefore happiness—as well as healthier foods. You choose those foods without a shred of guilt if you really need them or if the essential pain of not eating them is too great.

"The ribs and steaks aren't so important now . . . "

George's progress was slow but sure. With some reluctance, he learned to use the nurturing and limits cycles to soothe and calm himself so his fuse was not as short at work. He didn't launch into so many aggressive discussions, and his employees responded by being more cooperative. Plus they seemed to like him better.

His home life also improved. He opened up to Barbara about sensitive issues, such as his needing to feel more a part of the family and less of an outsider. Barbara felt relieved that George was finally talking about what was really bothering him.

George was less direct with the boys. He spent more time with Josh, the younger of the two, who was eager for his dad's attention, but Ben, the teenager, was more aloof. George normally would have pressed Ben, but with better limits, he let Ben take his own time to warm up again.

And George was eating in a balanced way naturally. Ribs and steaks just weren't that important to him now. Besides, he had to keep his food light in the evening to have energy to play ball with the boys. It seemed that George's weight solution was beginning to take hold.

It was balancing her moods that helped Stacy the most.

Although Stacy had tried before to eat only when she was hungry, the strategy had never worked, because her emotional drives were so strong that her eating felt beyond her control. By using the method, that is, mastering the six cures, she became aware of her feelings throughout the day and could tame them with the limits cycle. Her emotional roller coasters, and the compulsive eating that accompanied them, dwindled.

For instance, she could maintain emotional balance even after an encounter with an angry customer that previously would have triggered a candy bar binge. Now she could pause, still aware of the angry customer, and use the nurturing cycle: "I feel afraid. I need to protect myself. Would you please accept my apology?" Then tame those feelings by using the limits cycle: "I expect to apologize, but not to be abused. Just because I made a mistake doesn't mean I'm incompetent. Sometimes things go wrong and customers are angry. That's life." Stacy could then relax and deal with the crisis, still maintaining her emotional balance and feeling little need for a candy bar.

Stacy also "fired" her doctor and found another who would listen to her and help her with her PMS. Last, she accepted her body build, determining that a few pounds up or down the scale didn't really matter. Her rounded hips were in some ways sensual and comforting. Stacy felt tremendously relieved that she could now pass along her body pride to her daughter.

As she solved her weight problem, Stacy occasionally overate, but it didn't bother her, because she knew that since she had quieted the mind-body drives to overeat, the next day she would naturally eat less. Most important, she felt physically vital and emotionally balanced for the first time.

Taking a five-mile run every day is *not* mastery living.

The lifestyle so many of us face is two-dimensional: work and food. Surely sleep, love and relaxation factor into this way of life, but often the sum total of the week doesn't add up to as much fulfillment as we desire.

When life borders on depletion, food often takes center stage as the primary source of gratification, relief, soothing and reward. *Dieting becomes impossible.* When food has become *that* central to our gratification, tampering with it can trigger scarcity panics, dig-in-your-heels stubbornness or outright revolts, all which express themselves by eating ravenously.

Mastery Living, the last of the six cures, involves reshaping our lifestyles to ensure that they bring fulfillment and health, so that food is only one small part of the pleasure and fulfillment of the day.

Am I physically active?

Weight loss studies show over and over again that the best insurance against regaining weight is to exercise. Name the ben-

Cure 6. Mastery Living

An active and fulfilling lifestyle.

3. Time to Restore

1. Exercise

2. Meaningful Activities

efits of exercise and the list is long, but the real impact probably isn't so much the calories burned—it takes fifteen minutes of exercise to expend the energy in a measly little apple—but the effect of increased calorie loss after exercise (thermogenesis), the beefing up of calorie-burning muscle and the way exercise douses the emotional fires of overeating.

For many, the mental dividend physical activity pays is an overriding effect, as it takes away the urge for afternoon chips and bedtime ice cream. Receiving the full body-mind benefits of physical activity for a weight solution means exercising for *at least* thirty minutes every day.

On the other hand, excessive exercise has been linked to increased rates of mortality and may spin one's lifestyle out of balance so that other needs go unmet. Moreover, excessive exercise can be a way of camouflaging an emotional overeating difficulty that exercising can't completely resolve. On the average, a balanced exercise program of thirty to ninety minutes a day is optimal for most of us.

Am I engaging in meaningful activities?

Life is inherently anxiety provoking. Overeating and being inactive are two ways of coping with that anxiety. Engaging in meaningful activities is another. Pursuits we see as worthy can take us out of ourselves and away from anxiety as quickly and thoroughly as a cheeseburger or a cookie, but without a trace of weight gain.

Self-awareness is essential, but at some point that self-focus can be excessive. When all we can see is *our* feelings, *our* thoughts and *our* needs, the world becomes dreary and we become . . . more anxious!

Rabbi Hillel asks, "If I am not for myself, who will be? If I am only for myself, what am I?" Of course, he is right. A calming effect occurs when that self-focus is balanced by an other focus. That attention to giving rather than taking enables us to look back on the day and say to ourselves, "See, *I* did that. That *means* something!" Television, empty chatter and superficial activities lose our interest in comparison to the charge we get from doing something that *matters*.

What are meaningful pursuits? Whatever you feel is a contribution that matters: listening patiently to a friend, volunteering in a school, becoming politically active, reading to a small child. In short, *anything* that lifts you out of an overfocus on yourself and settles you down with a sense of the noble.

Am I taking time to restore myself?

The last part of the mastery living cycle is taking time each day to restore inner balance in mind and body. It is the devoted practice of setting aside time each day to refill the well inside, rather than solely taking from it.

Just the way engaging in meaningful pursuits gives something of you to the world, taking time to restore gives something of you back to yourself. And you need this, for too much meaningful activity can become a problem in and of itself.

Typically, restoring ourselves requires time to *rest, reflect, express* and *create*. It is time devoted to pleasures that indulge us without harm: a walk on the beach, picking flowers in the garden, sinking into a hot tub, sumptuous lovemaking or putting your feet up and taking a snooze. When and how you restore yourself is very individual, but the cornerstone of mastering this is becoming a devoted caretaker of yourself.

> *Stacy enjoyed antiques and aerobics; George chose chess and soccer.*

By the time Stacy and George had accomplished the other cures, they were already naturally creating lives for themselves that were active, meaningful and restoring.

George was playing soccer with his kids, took up chess with Ben, who was now feeling closer to his dad, and was renewed by both his friendship and his sensual life with Barbara. Weight and food were no longer problems—he had lost eighteen pounds and the doctor said he didn't need blood pressure medication.

With fewer mood swings and more energy, Stacy's life became balanced, with time for antiques hunting with Thomas, aerobics classes with friends and writing in her journal before breakfast. Life was good, and the weight problem that had gripped her for so long was over.

You can do this . . .

George and Stacy are not different from you and me. They had their difficulties and their reluctances. They used this method with neither an obsessive fervor nor a careless attitude, but in the manner they would use to address an imperfect but important task.

Today their weight problems are solved. Their lives are still full of hassles and demands, yet George and Stacy say they are more vibrant, fulfilled and happy than they have ever been. What's more, they don't feel compelled to step on the scale each morning, count the fat grams in all their food or chastise themselves whenever they overeat. In a sense, both George and Stacy are finally free.

A Simple Pathway to a Profound Cure

In this chapter, you will find everything you need to retrace the steps that led to your weight problem, so you can walk away from it forever.

Simply knowing how you got where you are now and then seeing the path to ending your weight problem will be a huge relief, leaving you ready to master the method at your own pace and in your own way.

I can vividly recall my confusion about my eating and weight. How did I acquire this curse? What was "wrong" with me? I had no idea how to resolve my weight issues, in part, because I didn't know how I developed them! I hope this chapter will relieve any of this kind of confusion you might have and bring you a sense of calm and clarity about how you will resolve your weight problem.

How does a weight solution happen?

There are four steps that lead to a weight problem. Solving a weight problem takes retracing those same four steps.

As I describe the eight stages of a weight problem, you'll meet two of my patients, Anne and Kevin, a married couple whose story is typical of those who master the method.

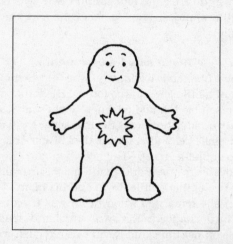

At one point, there was balance.

There was a time in your life when you had no trace of a weight problem, neither the weight itself nor the steps that led to it. You were in balance: your needs were met most of the time and you were aware of the strength, wisdom and goodness inside you. It is important that you recall when that might have been— whether it was only during your first moments of life, extended through early childhood or lasted into the adolescent or adult years. It is a semblance of that *state of balance* to which you will return when your weight problem is solved.

Anne was the adored child . . .

Anne, a 30-year-old woman with red hair and an infectious laugh, was raised in a family in which money was scarce. There were five children, and her mother sometimes drank too much but managed to keep the family going. Her father was away a lot, but showered the family with love when he returned. The biggest hugs were saved for Anne, who was his favorite. "You are the prettiest girl in the world," he'd say as he swung her around and tickled her.

As she grew older and could see that her mother was overwhelmed by the needs of the other children, Anne helped her and relished the role. Anne had a cheerful manner, and being the oldest child, she was adored by her brothers and sisters. In fact, she was the jewel of the family.

Kevin was less fortunate.

Anne's husband, Kevin, who was 39 when I met him, was not at all the jewel of his family. His father, whom he greatly resembled, had died when Kevin was 3. Although he had two older brothers, Kevin's sensitive nature and crooked smile reminded his mother of her beloved husband, so at first he received all her attention. Although the other boys were there and made noise, in reality it was just the two of them, little Kevin and his mom.

Then she remarried when Kevin was 6 years old and the picture changed. Her new husband made many demands on her time, and Kevin was often left with baby-sitters and neighbors or left alone to watch television.

Despite the demands of her situation, Anne had been in balance for much of her childhood, whereas Kevin had had only a brief honeymoon of inner harmony for his first few years. At present, Kevin could not recall ever feeling balanced. Yet he had been, because like all of us, he had had an innate sense of his own wisdom, strength and goodness at one time in his life. All of us have experienced a period of inner balance—even if it was only in the womb.

When was the time earlier in life when you felt in balance?

Stage 1. Few Skills

Stage 1 occurs in the early years and lays the groundwork for a weight problem to develop, not because of what happens, but because of *what does not*. During this time, we need our parents to give us enough skill in the six cures to sustain us through the challenges life will hold for us. But through no fault of our own, we don't acquire enough of these skills to give us the vital protection and resilience we will need.

How much is *enough*? The challenges vary for each of us, depending upon our choices and fate. However, in order to quiet the initial rumblings of a weight problem we require *higher levels* of these skills if we have *higher levels* of:

- External stress—the stresses life holds, including losses, changes and traumas

- Internal stress—an internal temperament that is difficult to manage, particularly in the areas of high sensitivity, strong emotions, a tendency to withdraw and body signals that are difficult to interpret

- Genetic weight problems—a genetic tendency to gain weight in a society that has few built-in sources of exercise and taunts us with an overabundance of delectable foods

In retrospect, there is little confusion about whether or not you received enough of these skills. By definition, if your weight is above your genetic comfort zone, you *did not* receive as much of these skills as you needed given your circumstances.

Perhaps the most convincing way to lock into your thinking that the skills you received were low is to reflect on your experience growing up:

- Were you secure in knowing that your *separate* feelings and needs were important and valued and comfortable that you could ask for help?

- Were the limits set for you appropriate for *the person you were* at that time—neither too difficult nor too easy?

- Were you taught that your body was sacred and worthy, your health important and that the vitality of your lifestyle mattered?

How hard your parents tried or what their personal impediments to parenting were is *not* the issue. Their responsibility in raising you wasn't just to take you to the requisite number of ball games, put three meals on the table and plan your birthday parties. These signposts of adequate parenting are not very meaningful. You were not a nameless, faceless "generic" child but a unique individual in need of being given exactly what you needed to master the six cures. It was their job to shape their parenting so that the *result* was your mastery of the six cures. For example, the child with:

- Genetic obesity needs extra help in developing positive attitudes about eating fruit or playing soccer.

- A sensitive temperament needs more guidance in setting limits as a protection from life's woes.

- Unusual stresses, such as a parent who is distant, needs license to express the whole range of emotions to heal that hurt.

Is this completely unrealistic? Yes and no.

Yes, because these cures aren't just parenting skills, they are the hidden *intimate processes* that form the foundation of how we parent. Therefore, the daughter who adopted the harsh inner voice of her depriving parents during childhood can read stacks of advice books on parenting. Even if she "acts the part"—using positive discipline and giving loving back rubs—it isn't enough. For as long as her inner life is judgmental and not nurturing, the child will adopt the same critical inner voice. Likewise, she may have reasonable expectations for her children—yet retain harsh ones for herself. The result? The child mirrors her parent and sets the same impossibly high standards for herself.

No, because a surprising number of children have parents with substantial amounts of these skills and they don't develop weight problems despite stresses and a tendency to put on extra pounds. What the rest of us struggle to learn as adults, these children have achieved by the age of 6. This is a matter of fate, which asks for our acceptance. However, we must take up the baton where our parents left off and give ourselves *every measure* of the skills we need. By doing so we become heroes, for we have stopped the flow of these patterns from one generation to the next.

Anne needed few of these skills at first.

As her mom's best friend and substitute companion while her father was away, Anne was treated as a peer by her mother, who set few explicit limits. Interestingly, the family's lifestyle was such that there was little need for internal limits. School days and even weekend activities

The Stages of a Weight Problem

A Weight Problem Begins . . .

Stage 1. Few Skills

We don't have enough of the skills needed to protect our health and happiness.

Stage 2. Distress Mounts

Without enough protection, problems arise and distress mounts.

Stage 3. Balance Is Lost

Our inner life stops being a safe and soothing place to go. We lose our inner balance and begin to seek external solutions to our distress.

Stage 4. External Solutions

We use external solutions to our distress, including overeating and inactivity. A weight problem develops.

A Weight Problem Is Solved . . .

Stage 5. Less Distress

We use the Thinking Journals and Feelings Letters to decrease our distress.

Stage 6. More Skills

We master the six cures and become more effective at protecting our health and happiness.

Stage 7. Balance Is Restored

Our inner life becomes a safe and soothing place to go. We regain our inner balance and begin to seek internal solutions to our distress.

Stage 8. Internal Solutions

External solutions are no longer as necessary. Eating and activity are often balanced and weight decreases and stays within its genetic comfort zone.

were highly scheduled, and because the food budget was tight, the milk was watered, snacks and second helpings were unheard of and cookies appeared only at Christmas. Moreover, Anne was active in sports like basketball, swimming and volleyball and was used to strict practice schedules that kept her busy and away from food.

Although austere, her home life was reasonably nurturing, so she was emotionally content. All in all, with the combination of some skills of her own in the six cures and a family life that filled in where her skills fell short, Anne stayed in reasonable balance for the first two and a half decades of her life. However, during this time the clock was ticking. Although she didn't know it, because her skills were few, the ground was laid for a full-blown weight problem.

Kevin learned that all limits were harsh ones.

Anne's husband, Kevin, has vivid memories of his stepfather, Paul. A career military man, Paul was hard on Kevin, and after he arrived on the scene when Kevin was 6, he set about toughening him up. He took Kevin's older brothers camping, fishing and hunting. However, because Kevin had severe allergies, he couldn't run or go on outdoor adventures. Paul scoffed at Kevin's allergies and implied that he was weak and inadequate. Further, Paul insisted that his wife stop treating Kevin "like a baby," so she withheld tenderness and warmth.

Kevin began to feel totally alone. He was an outsider to the three males in the family, and his mother, exhausted from work and disappointment in her second marriage, seemed to be in another world. Family meals were excruciating to Kevin. His mother sulked, Paul reprimanded the boys on table manners, and his brothers acted like hoodlums, shouting and laughing and making mischief. Kevin withdrew from it all and soothed himself with what was on his plate.

How much skill in the six cures did you gain growing up?
How much more did you acquire as an adult?

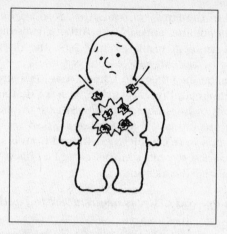

Stage 2. Distress Mounts

At some point, the demands of life overwhelm our ability to deal with them. A backlog of unresolved feelings, what I call emotional trash, starts piling up. As it does, we enter the second stage of a weight problem. Once the losses, hurts and stresses enter our inner life they tend to stay there because we do not have the skill to become aware of our disappointments and feel the essential pain involved, thereby releasing the hurt.

We experience this buildup of distress as tension, anger, sadness, fear and numbness, and being rational and sane we want to flee from it. With our attention turned toward a way to escape, our awareness of ourselves wanes and it becomes increasingly hard to see ourselves as worthy and life as good.

The emotional trash keeps us from drawing on our own innate wisdom, strength and goodness. Our inner self, once a sanctuary for soothing and comforting ourselves, begins to seem empty or even threatened. We grow afraid to venture inside ourselves—and the less we venture inside, the more unfriendly our inner life becomes.

The amount of distress inside Kevin was far greater than that within Anne.

Both Anne and Kevin had difficulty pinpointing when their distress began to mount. In the end, Anne realized that she had minimized the influence of the special role she held in the family of being the "good" girl and care-taker of her mother and siblings. Although she didn't have a weight problem until her mid-20's, the distress was mounting by her early adolescent years.

Kevin, on the other hand, knew that his distress must have begun mounting early in life, with the double trauma of the loss of his father and the entry into his life of a rejecting stepfather. What perplexed Kevin was that his observations were completely detached from his feelings. When he tried to reflect on his early life, his mind went blank. All he felt was numb.

At what age did distress begin mounting within you?

Stage 3. Balance Is Lost

This mounting distress feels like layers and layers of the kinds of feelings that we'd all rather avoid. Our inner life is no longer a soothing and comforting sanctuary, and we are in a quandary, for our choices are few.

We can choose to feel all the feelings mounting inside us—not just the pleasurable ones but the distressing ones, too. Or we can stop feeling entirely. If we chose to feel, thereby opening the spigot to an inner life, all the pent-up feelings—not just the pleasurable ones—will seep out or gush out against our will.

As a result, there comes a time, the third stage of a weight problem, when too much emotional distress has mounted within, and we close ourselves off from our inner life, simply out of expediency. *We can't take it anymore.* Cut off from our inner wisdom, strength and goodness, we can no longer find our emotional balance.

In Kevin's life, football was the last straw.

Kevin's balance had been lost for some time, and his way of coping was to withdraw from everyone, do his homework and watch hours and hours of television. He became a quiet and introverted boy who was increasingly pudgy from his lack of exercise and preoccupation with solitary pursuits.

Yet right after his twelfth birthday, a shot at playing football stirred Kevin's imagination, and he took it upon himself to lift weights and take up running so he could make the team. Paul encouraged Kevin, and for a few months they actually became closer. Sadly, Kevin encountered a football coach during tryouts who laughed him off the playing field by saying he was far too fat and too slow to have a prayer of making the team. Even more dreadful, Paul turned on his stepson, agreed with the coach and blamed Kevin for watching too much television and being too greedy with food.

As he looked back on it during one of our sessions, Kevin said that he saw that moment as the turning point. It was then that what remained of emotional balance was lost. He cut the cord to his inner life because when he went inside all he could hear was his stepfather's judgmental voice. Kevin looked for a better alternative for comfort than his own inner life and, as it turned out, the one he chose was food.

His high school years were a blur. He was a whiz at math, and studied accounting in college. While at college, he met Anne. They hit it off immediately, though it was Anne who did the initial pursuing. "He was a big bear of a man, like my father. The night I met him he looked so lonely and defeated, I just wanted to hug him." Anne laughed. "I haven't stopped hugging him since." Kevin couldn't believe his good fortune. They married while still in college, then moved to San Francisco. They both joined a big accounting firm. Kevin was in the tax department and Anne took a position in human resources.

A new baby, a new home, a new distress . . .

Anne's life at college was scheduled down to the last midterm, the last volleyball match and the last meal of the day. She was on a scholarship, and wanted to keep it.

When she met Kevin her life felt perfect. He was quiet, sweet and so grateful for all her attention.

Their move to San Francisco and working at the accounting firm were all a great adventure, and her life continued to be very structured but pleasurable. Breakfast was before 8:00 A.M., lunch was shared with Kevin at noon and dinner was after her workout at the gym, usually around 8:00 P.M. Anne recalls that she loved the human resources department and found she had a knack for choosing the right person for a particular job. Kevin progressed well in the tax department, and there was talk of bringing him into the partnership. Life was good.

Three years later Kevin was made a partner in the firm, and Anne discovered she was pregnant. With his six-figure salary, they purchased a new house in the Berkeley hills where there were lots of families. Their life had gone so smoothly that neither Kevin nor Anne could have expected what followed. Anne came home from the hospital with their little baby, Brittany, to a life of isolation, inner turmoil and utter chaos.

For Anne, the external controls of the regimented life vanished.

It was tax season and Anne hardly saw Kevin. She was left to adjust to a total lack of structure in her personal life and no professional structure to guide her either. Moreover, she felt like a social recluse. She didn't know anyone in the neighborhood, and with the endless demands of the baby, she was too tired and depressed to knock on doors and start making new friends. Anne felt entirely alone.

Kevin was working harder now to make up for the loss of a second income, and was often physically or emotionally absent. All the attention he used to get from Anne was now going to the baby.

In addition, Anne seemed different. She was so worried about him overworking that it was a constant issue between them. She often gave Kevin unasked-for advice about how he could manage his work better. He resented her intrusiveness and protected himself by sharing less information with her. Even though he was surrounded by clients and colleagues all day, Kevin felt at least as isolated as Anne.

When did your inner life stop being a safe and soothing place to go?

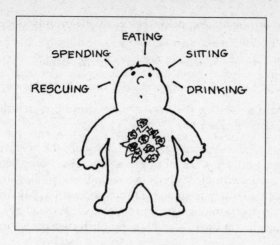

Stage 4. External Solutions

As our distress mounts, what do we do? We do what any intelligent person would do when going inside themselves is no longer safe. We go *outside,* thus beginning the fourth stage of a weight problem.

Not only have we severed our connection to the wisdom, strength and goodness inside us, but unwittingly we've taken on a whole host of new problems. Without that inner resource to draw upon, one innocuous slice of chocolate fudge cake becomes a slab of cake and then another. A few evenings on the couch watching videos slide into weeks without any exercise whatsoever. And we become vulnerable to other subtle or blatant shifts in our actions, whether it be in work, love, money or addictive substances.

What's more, our progress in mastering the six cures ceases. Just the way we can't build upper body strength without moving our arms and shoulders, we cannot beef up our skills in the six cures without tapping into our inner life. When we close the door on our inner life, we stay locked into patterns that don't work for us, advancing in years but not in our effectiveness in dealing with life's challenges.

What do we do to externally gratify, soothe and distract ourselves? *It doesn't really matter.* We could:

- Overeat, overdrink, overspend, overwork, overexercise or oversit

- Take drugs, smoke, drive recklessly, be promiscuous or intentionally fail

- Please people, rescue people or control people

- Escape into self-pity, depression, rages or fantasies

- Present a sociable demeanor to the world but isolate ourselves emotionally

They are all essentially the same. They are the best we can do at the time, but they are all external solutions. Some people find one external solution, such as overeating, and stick with it for a lifetime. Others skip from one solution to another, say from over-working to overdrinking to overexercising, or keep a bevy of small excesses going at once, so no one problem ever draws too much attention.

All these patterns share a common function—to help us escape the inner abyss, the darkness or the anxiety. Unfortunately, that distraction blocks us from our own maturation.

This is where we move into a realm that inadvertently takes us further from our inner balance. This is the frightening part because even though we are out of balance and grasping for exter-nal solutions, those solutions have yet to become entrenched. We would readily slip back into balance given a slice of good fortune. Yet we often don't, because the lure of the external solution pulls us in that direction.

Unfortunately, the external solution creates more distress and a greater pile of emotional trash. Often it becomes a magnet for our attention—either feeling guilty about continuing it or trying to stop it. We have no reserves of mental or emotional energy to attend to the roots of the problem, where our true power to resolve it lies. The pattern persists, and a weight problem develops.

Anne went right to food . . .

After the baby was born, it took only a short time for Anne to seek an external solution. She might not have slipped so quickly and so far if she had not been alone and so tired from the physical demands of little Brittany.

Kevin seemed happy with the baby, and Anne didn't want to become the stereotypical homemaker who com-plained every time she opened her mouth. So she with-drew and said nothing, and that was when she began to sink into a depression. The malaise lasted six years—until she began using the method.

Why did she fall into patterns of overeating? There is no way of knowing, but when I asked Anne, she responded, "Food was scarce in my family. There was not always enough to go around, so of course I didn't overeat. Later, when I needed some external comfort, it only made sense to choose something that held special meaning to me."

The other external solution Anne adopted was rescuing others—assuming the responsibility for fixing problems that were beyond her authority to resolve. "I was accustomed to taking care of my mother without her really knowing it," Anne said. "I was used to doing the behind-the-scenes work of making the family life smooth. I never thought that meddling in his life was disrespectful. I considered it my job to do it."

Kevin hit the candy machine and worked incessantly.

Kevin was brutally frank about the external solutions he found himself using. Food wasn't that important in his family. However, the abrupt loss of his dad, the intense overinvolvement with his mother followed by the loss of his mother's devotion and the punishing, critical presence of Paul created a tug-of-war that left him confused and empty. Early in life, the sweetness of food and fullness of the belly constituted about the only choice available to him.

When Kevin spoke to me briefly about his overworking, he recognized that it fulfilled his need to gain his boss's favor. It wasn't simply a matter of securing his job, but a deeper need that reverberated with his dissatisfying relationship with Paul. According to Kevin, "Even though it's irrational, there is a drive in me to please him at all costs, and when I do please him, it gives me a disproportionate amount of pleasure. I see that now, but initially, I just thought of myself as a diligent worker. But the drive is far more compelling than a normal work drive."

At what age did you begin to seek external solutions?

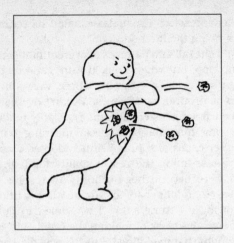

Stage 5. Less Distress

To turn a weight problem around requires going back inside. But before we can do that we have to make the inner environment safe again.

Thus the fifth stage of a weight problem is to do some emotional housecleaning. This is the stage of intentionally lightening the emotional backlog of tension, distress and numbness within. Most of our emotional trash won't voluntarily emerge. In fact it hides from us in curious ways. We may:

- Develop a huge appetite that is an expression of our anger or fear

- Paralyze ourselves with depression rather than feel the sadness

- Feel lethargic or become sick without understanding why

- Stay incessantly busy to fend off emotions

- Laugh when a situation is sad or grin when we are angry

- Be rather unemotional, then weep at any movie that is at all sad

- Have a chip on our shoulder

- Act exceedingly nice, then fly into rages

- Act removed or elated when things have gone terribly wrong

Of course, there are many ways to release distress, but in this method we use a very direct approach: Thinking Journals and Feelings Letters. The journals bring up the thoughts that you least want to think but most need to think if your life is to get better. The letters create a structure for releasing the feelings these thoughts elicit. When used together these can be very powerful tools.

There are fourteen journals in the method and as many letters as you need to release the feelings these journals arouse. The journals build upon one another to enable you to release past hurts, return to emotional balance and make your life become even better.

Anne was hesitant.

Anne took several weeks to get around to writing the journals. That was fine, as everyone goes at their own pace along the path.

"I found that eating a small pepperoni pizza while reading the evening newspaper and watching my favorite sitcom on television was far easier than writing the journals. But I knew that focusing on Kevin's work troubles and my own dieting didn't make either problem better, so finally I got my courage up and wrote the first journal. I was afraid it would leave me dangling emotionally.

"I was afraid that if I thought about everything that's happened, it would depress me for days. Perhaps it would have, but I wrote a Feelings Letter to my mother, and another to myself. They took me a whole hour to write, but I felt so much better, like a weight was off my shoulders. The technique is much more effective than I expected."

Anne wrote the journals and the letters slowly, one set of them each week. The nurturing journal brought up a lot of pain for Anne, but she survived it. She was actually becoming skilled at sitting with the pain, knowing that it would go away, rather than running from the pain by putting food into her mouth. The later journals that helped Anne face her aloneness and carve out a new vision of herself were the most transforming to her, and after writing them her weight began to drop quite a bit. In fact, one week she lost three pounds and the next, to her surprise, another two without being aware she was eating less. I noticed in class that Anne looked thinner and her face had spontaneous freshness that probably came from both the internal changes she was orchestrating and the way her lifestyle had changed because of it.

Kevin plunged into healing.

Kevin was more than ready to unload some of his distress. He attacked the journals, writing one a day until he was done—then wrote every one of them a second time. Although this would be far too intense for some people, it was just what Kevin needed.

"I wanted to get the past off my back. I wrote about my stepfather, my mother, my brothers, and what a worm I was to take that crap from them then and from my boss now. I wrote about 50 Feelings Letters the first two months of the program. When it came to the later journals, the ones in which I look at my own life and what I want from it, I was ready to seriously think about it for the first time in my life. I wasn't on autopilot anymore."

When will you begin lessening your distress?

Stage 6. More Skills

The sixth stage of a weight problem is to boost your skills in the six cycles of the method. In Part 4 of this book, The Six Cure Records will give you added structure to master them. Once you have the skills in hand, you'll be prepared to take care of your health and happiness even when external circumstances are far from ideal.

There is no doubt you can master the cures. Just the way you learned a way of operating that didn't keep you in balance, you can learn a way that does. In any case, it's not as if you are starting at *ground zero*. You already have some or a lot of these skills; all you are doing now is enhancing them.

Kevin's needs had long gone unmet. The six cures changed that.

With more personal drive than he had ever known, Kevin lit into mastering the six cures. He visited me every other week and was definitely focused. He wanted to master the method and he wanted to do it now.

That's just what he did. Kevin started not with the

nurturing cycle, but with the limits cycle. He was a thought-oriented person, and it was easier for him to be aware of his thoughts than his feelings. Interestingly, once he used the limits cure, his focus automatically switched to feelings, so he restored inner balance in his own way.

The body cures were easy for Kevin because he was healthy and his body size was never an issue for him. But he did find a good doctor and began screening for cholesterol and blood pressure, as well as attending to a few skin problems that had bothered him.

Moreover, he realized how much his body pride had suffered since his intimate life with Anne had all but vanished when Brittany was born. Before he gained these skills he would not have talked with Anne about sex, because it would have turned into a yelling match. But now Kevin did bring up the subject and was able to talk with Anne in a loving yet assertive way.

It turned out that Anne had so many weightist thoughts that she assumed Kevin was not attracted to her heavier body. Kevin told her, "Anne, I fell in love with you, not just the size of your body. If you weigh more, that doesn't change the fact I'm excited by you."

Kevin changed his work schedule and set a limit to be home by 7:30 P.M., after stopping off at the gym on his way. He had always loved television, and meat and potatoes dinners, but these no longer satisfied him. It wasn't that he didn't enjoy a big steak or an evening on the couch, but his time with Anne and Brittany had become so meaningful to him that heavy dinners and evenings zoned out watching TV lost their appeal.

For Anne, life was exciting again, and the layers of weight began to come off.

Strong Nurturing jump-started Anne's weight solution. She needed that sense of letting go of everyone and everything and just paying attention to herself. Still, it was a little unsettling. It was easy for her to know how everyone else felt. Her own feelings were so confusing that she often didn't know how she felt.

Effective Limits made her more realistic about what she could accomplish. Could she really expect herself to be isolated and take care of a baby all day, have no adult emotional and intellectual stimulation, yet not want to eat everything in sight? No. So Anne began to feed herself in ways other than eating. She joined a gym that had infant care, and wanted to go back to work part time. Eventually she started a small company out of her home, which referred English nannies to affluent San Franciscans. She began to enjoy herself again.

She also let go of intruding on Kevin's life after realizing that trying to solve Kevin's problems was disrespectful to him. How could she be sexually attracted to a man she felt she had to mother? Kevin was an adult, not her child, and he had his own supply of wisdom with which to manage his problems.

Besides, she had to take care of her own health and happiness. Sinking into self-pity and powerlessness was something she didn't have to do anymore. The earth was not going to fall in if she gained fifty pounds, so using weight as a way of saying "Help me! Feel sorry for me!" was both childish and pointless.

Anne felt her old excitement coming back and found herself feeling more affectionate toward Kevin. The joking and laughing they had both treasured before Brittany arrived began to return. Life was busier and more exciting, just the way Anne liked it, and there was still time for her daughter.

"I feel great and sad at the same time," Anne admitted to me. "If I had just learned the six cures earlier I wouldn't have wasted all that time being miserable. All I had to do was know what I was feeling and follow through in meeting my needs. You can bet I'm teaching my kids how to express themselves, too. I just love it when Brittany comes up to me and says, 'Mommy, I need a hug.'"

When will you begin taking better care of your health and happiness?

Stage 7. Balance Is Restored

This method is not about fairy tales and life miraculously turning into Utopia. It's all about balance. Even when our inner life becomes safe again and we become more skilled at finding internal solutions to our distress, life is far from perfect.

You will still bump into emotional trash when you go inside. But you will be able to be with your feelings, and you will be skilled at expressing them rather than riding roughshod over them, burying them deeper. You can soothe and comfort yourself from within, even though your inner life is not a clean slate. In fact, those remnants from your personal history are something to take pride in, proof that you have evolved and matured.

The minister at St. John's Church in Ross, California, Bart Sarjeant, once said to me when I was feeling a great deal of pain, "Laurel, the tragedies of life are like leaves on a tree. They fall to the ground, and when they do, they nourish the tree and make it stronger." In a similar way, the residue of past losses and hurts can enrich your inner balance just as the patina of old sterling silver is far more pleasing to the eye than the bright shininess of the new.

Although reconnecting with one's inner life sounds like a somber experience, many people find it electrifying and joyful. My patients say:

> *"I feel so intense and so present. It is almost like a drug except better. It is real!"*

> *"Can I keep this up? I don't want to go back to how I was, but my whole day feels different. Everything is bright and real feeling."*

A deeper transformation is occurring. Individuals grab hold of life with reverence and exuberance and the intense excitement of possessing themselves perhaps for the first time. And it shows. Friends, neighbors, co-workers and relatives notice the difference. There is a new spontaneity and a fascinating vibrancy about them—all reflections of the balance in the mind, body and spirit—that is very dramatic.

Kevin's journey was unusually fast . . .

Kevin was so ripe for change when he began using the method that he was inordinately quick to reclaim his inner balance.

I knew he had reached the seventh stage when he stopped coming to our individual sessions. He canceled two visits in a row, and the second time he called to cancel, we talked about it.

Kevin said, "I don't know why, but I don't want to come to the session."

I replied, "Well, let's figure out what it is. Do you have any ideas?"

Kevin paused, then replied, "It's just that I have so much going on . . . "

"Work?"

"No. Not my work. I set a limit with work and that's been good. It's the rest of my life. I'm feeling really impatient because there is so much I want to do. I've pretty much talked Anne into a trip to England this spring. I've always loved England, and I realized, if I like it so much, why wasn't I going there? And Brittany and Allison have their soccer teams and I don't want to miss their game and I haven't had a problem with weight really. I lose a pound or two a week and that overeating I did before? I don't have the desire anymore . . . "

It was clear to me then that Kevin had mastered the method. Once he had those developmental skills under his belt, he didn't need me. In fact, time spent at our sessions would only hold him back.

Anne needed to pause along the way.

Anne required more time and took a less direct route.

In fact, she told the group in frustration, "How come I don't get it yet? Why is my progress so slow? Yes, I'm changing, but not like Kevin. Kevin's so different now and I feel like he's leaving me in the dust, that I'm just not keeping up."

Another group member who has become a friend of Anne's spoke up: "Anne, I know you. You're my friend and I know why it's slower for you. You still don't like going inside or you don't do it as often. You are so used to numbing out on food that checking in with your feelings and thoughts is strange and foreign to you. I don't see why you are so hard on yourself. You're on the right road, and it may take longer, but everybody's journey has its own pace. You don't have to be like Kevin. Just relax into it. Please."

For the next few weeks Anne allowed herself to relax and submitted to the program more, not worrying about her results, just concentrating on going inside and using the cures. About a month after she shared her worries with the group, Anne came to the session glowing. "I'm not like Kevin and I didn't have such a monumental conversion, but I'm definitely feeling different. It's working and I know it is because this week we had major disasters at home and work, yet I didn't want the snack I usually have late in the evening. In fact, I lost two pounds in one week and I wasn't even dieting. In my own way, I think I'm back in balance. I feel more content than I can ever remember feeling. I don't have to run here and there and do too much and take care of everybody all the time. At times, I can just 'be' and that is enough."

When do you expect that your balance will be restored?

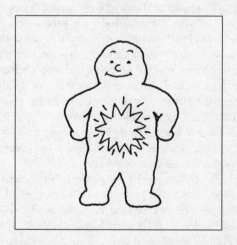

Stage 8. Internal Solutions

The last stage of a weight problem is the easiest. The roots of the weight problem have been clipped, and the leaves from the tree fall naturally. The excessive appetites, such as overeating and inactivity, come less often, and in their place are reasonably—but not perfectly—healthy patterns. When you do overeat or fall away from your exercise program, it doesn't matter. You can—at your own pace—regain balance and return to healthier patterns.

It's as if the moment of the weight problem has passed, the drama is over and the weight problem is gone. Moreover, you are more alive, more vibrant and more peaceful than you were in the beginning. This balance in mind, body and lifestyle that was your birthright, you have personally and finally reclaimed.

Waving good-bye to your weight problem . . .

Anne and Kevin were subjects in our testing of the method, and they came to my home on a Saturday several months later so I could collect data for the study and so we could all catch up with each other. Both of them looked vibrant and happy. Anne had lost twenty-three pounds by then and Kevin had dropped eighteen.

They were full of information about their lives: the trip to England was next month, Brittany had started horse-back-riding lessons and Kevin had received a new assignment at work, which amounted to a promotion, despite the limits he had put on his work hours. Anne was taking a night class at the college in sculpture and priming her business to open a second office in the next county.

Later, as I walked them out to their car, I told Anne and Kevin how happy I was for them. Anne responded, "It's not just that I've lost twenty-three pounds. It's what I've found. I never knew I could be so strong and so happy. I know there are always problems, but I don't feel so devastated by the things that come up.

"I can't say that my eating is perfect, but I can say that it's very good, and I *don't care* that it's not perfect. I don't have to be perfect! My weight is down and I feel really healthy and strong and secure within myself. If I didn't have the weight problem, I never would have made these changes." She smiled. "So, I'm . . . content."

I gave her a hug. She and Kevin got into their car, and I watched them drive away, comforted by knowing that they had each solved their weight problem forever.

Now you have seen the pathway that Anne and Kevin walked, which is the same one that you can chose to take. It is not complex. Walking it requires the diligence to put one foot in front of the other, taking—at times—very small steps, writing the journals and letters and using the cures over and over again until they become part of your natural functioning.

The missing piece of the puzzle . . .

What may not be not clear from understanding the steps that lead to a weight solution is why using these very simple cures and writing these little journals and letters lead to such deep personal transformations.

It's because of the six unexpected rewards. In their own quiet, indirect way, the six rewards are the powerhouses that fuel these remarkable and lasting changes.

The Six Unexpected Rewards

Using these six basic skills that add to our personal resilience is *what we can do* to solve our weight problem. Yet something far more than these skills is the ultimate source of our weight solution.

It is the six unexpected rewards. These quiet inner changes come without any direct attention or personal effort on our part—other than consciously using the six cures. Yet their arrival is extraordinary and powerful.

Looking to the past for a moment, the havoc that the six causes wreaked was painful. Without the protection of the six cures, there may have been shadings of the consequences of inner chaos: emotional imbalance, a sense of impending peril, social isolation, personal lethargy and a profound feeling of emptiness.

These consequences are not fixed but quite fluid and through using the six cures changes appear. Instead of feeling divided and

---

What are the six unexpected rewards?

The six cures stimulate powerful, unexpected changes within: *the six rewards.*
These rewards then sustain your weight solution and change your life.

The Six Unexpected Rewards

Reward 1. Integration

The feeling of inner chaos will lessen. Seeing yourself as all good or all bad will be replaced by a sense of accepting yourself, imperfections and all. You will feel a more singular sense of who you are.

Reward 2. Balance

Emotional imbalance—the extreme highs and lows and numbness—will be replaced by a more positive and stable emotional life.

Reward 3. Sanctuary

The peril that comes from having no safe place inside to go will decrease. Instead, you will be aware of having a safe, loving sanctuary within, no matter what storms rage in your external life.

Reward 4. Intimacy

Isolation will be replaced by more intimacy. This is because you have a nurturing inner life that enhances openness and the limits to protect yourself from surrendering to another.

Reward 5. Vibrancy

Balanced eating, vigorous activity, body pride and optimal health will end lethargy and boost your body's vibrancy. You will look your best and feel radiant.

Reward 6. Spirituality

In time, the feelings of emptiness will lessen. In its place will come a renewed awareness of the goodness within you and a heightened appreciation for life's mystery and grace.

chaotic, we feel a sense of wholeness and integration. The impossible emotional highs, lows and numbness are superseded by a profound sense of balance. The peril is replaced by the experience of sanctuary, isolation by intimacy and lethargy by vibrancy. Finally, the emptiness is filled by a deeper appreciation of the spiritual nature of life.

The rewards come, even if we aren't perfect.

Marty called the week before Christmas, a year after she had completed training in the method. It was what she said to me that impressed me the most. If this woman who had more than her share of burdens could reap these six rewards, anyone could.

Marty's early life had been filled with tragedy. Both her parents had been killed in a car accident when she was 11. During her turbulent teen years, she bounced from sexual promiscuity to alcohol abuse to binge eating. As her weight increased, a congenital knee problem worsened and she endured two surgeries and much pain.

In time, Marty began to believe she could build something better in her life, and enrolled in a community college, aiming eventually to major in film production. She began working nights at the university computer center to support herself, saw an announcement about a Solution group starting and enrolled.

The first time I saw this 20-something woman with jet-black roots in her short white-blonde hair, I was struck by the intensity and toughness that only partially veiled her inner fragility. I could feel her pain and sensitivity and desperately wanted her to master the method and feel better. But I checked my own limits and held back from trying to "rescue" her. I purposely gave her the room she needed to take in the ideas of the method at her own pace and in her own way.

As it turned out, she participated in the session for only a few months, then left abruptly because of another round of knee surgery. Over time I lost track of her, as did her fellow group members. I worried about her. Then out of the blue, she called.

"Laurel, I'm doing great! So far I've lost fifty-two pounds, and it hasn't been hard. In fact, it has been incredibly easy. I never felt deprived, and I've made some other incredible changes too. You see . . ."

I felt a chill inside. "I'm listening, I'm listening."

"The nurturing worked great for me. I had to learn to honor my feelings and needs and that took time. Then I wanted some limits. The same ones I used to rebel against now seemed like the kind of protection I needed. Things went quickly from then on. My body felt healthier and the food wasn't that much of a problem. I started exercising because I enjoyed it, not because I was supposed to.

"I guess I was using the cures without being aware of it. About then I began to feel very different inside. The big ups, big downs and numbing myself didn't happen as often. I felt peaceful, and that's never happened to me before!

"My classes at college and work hassles stopped bothering me so much and I have a boyfriend now, someone who gives me love and treats me with respect. Mainly, I'm enjoying myself—and everything—more. It's strange because these things seemed to happen without me forcing them. Yes, it's great to be thinner—I can't wait for you to see me—but what's even more important to me is that my life is completely different. It is so much better."

When I hung up the phone after my conversation with Marty, I shuddered, remembering how these rather curious changes had also occurred in my own life when I solved my weight problem. I thought of many other patients who had told me of the identical experience. But it was an entirely different matter when I saw what these unexpected benefits had meant to Marty, who was so young and so burdened. If she could reap the rewards of the method, it must be powerful enough that others—using it imperfectly as we all do, burdened with the demands of life as we all are—could reap them too.

Once the inner journey begins, it has a life of its own.

Many of us have lived in an unbalanced way for years, riding an emotional roller coaster from extreme highs to abysmal lows, or sitting on the sidelines, feeling numb. We try to handle the upsets the world hands us by turning to external solutions—the cookies, the right job, the perfect love—until the solace we find inside ourselves is so satisfying and effective that continuing the inner journey becomes as unconscious and natural as breathing.

I first began to understand this from my friend Jim Billings, a psychologist and minister. The two of us were sitting in his office in Sausalito, which sits above the wharf filled with scruffy houseboats and looks out upon the sparkling hills of San Francisco beyond. He explained to me his view of the crossover between the mental and the spiritual. Leaning way back in his chair, and pausing the way people unconsciously do when they are about to say something that *really matters*, he said with a hush, "Once one begins the inner journey, that journey has a life of its own."

As Jim predicted, the rewards of reconnecting with the strength, wisdom and goodness within flow without our conscious effort. For many they trickle out slowly and imperceptibly. Often patients answer questions about their changes with the phrase "You know, it's funny, I've didn't think about it until now, but . . ." followed by a revelation of a completely dazzling change they have made in their life: the renewal of intimacy in a lifeless relationship, the release of other external solutions like drinking or smoking, a profound spiritual deepening or a growing interest in experiencing the bounties of life—like watching grizzly bears in Canada or fall leaves at their peak in New England.

For others, the changes are even more extreme. Rather than trickling out, the changes burst out like black gold from an oil well: the sudden and violent mourning of a parent lost during childhood, followed immediately by a sense of freedom and buoyancy; the strength, at last, to leave an abusive relationship; the courage to quit a dry, thankless career and train for a marvelous new one.

In honoring our inner life—our emotional, intellectual and spiritual base—we attain a clarity akin to the promise in the New Testament: "Consider the lilies of the field, how they grow; they neither toil nor spin; yet I tell you, even Solomon in all his glory was not arrayed like one of these."

Reward 1. Integration

The first unexpected reward of mastering the six cures is integration. The arrival of a feeling of wholeness and the departure of chaos are unmistakable.

Marsha was living with the pain of a dying husband, a beloved mother with Alzheimer's and a promotion at work that left her supervising an additional ten people in her accounting department. She found integration to be her most prized reward from mastering the method, far more important than the twenty-one pounds she lost.

"I've never had emotional problems, but I never felt solid, the way some of my friends do. I had to be overly good to my mother and husband, and on the job. Then there was the part of me that rebelled and ate whatever I wanted and stayed as big as I wanted to be. It was confusing because I didn't believe the good me and I felt ashamed of the bad me.

"I don't feel that way anymore. My being overweight is not so bad and my eating is just the part of me that acts rebellious. Doing so much for my husband, my mother and my staff wasn't good, it was foolish. Using the method got me to stop wanting to do everything for everyone except myself. I don't have to be perfectly virtuous anymore with my eating and weight or with other people. It feels so relaxing to be neither good nor bad, but just me."

When the two sides of ourselves make peace, our stress level plummets.

How and why does the method produce this sense of wholeness—of integration? It all starts with studies done on children and families, particularly the work of Salvador Minuchin, Hilde Bruch and Virginia Satir.

It appears that children must occupy a special place in the family to gain the warm acceptance, guidance and discipline they need to grow up reasonably balanced in mind, body and lifestyle. If they receive what they need from their parents and social milieu, they learn to treat themselves the same way they were treated and internalize the skills their parents model for them. In other words, they learn how to take care of their health and happiness.

The environment a child needs is illustrated in the diagram below. The child is in the child role and the parent is in the adult role. The line between them, called the *separation of the generations line*, is the invisible yet sacred line that allows children to be children.

The Child Is in a *Safe* Role

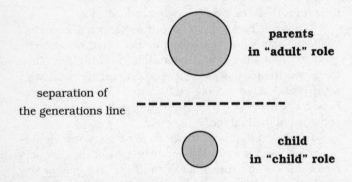

parents
in "adult" role

separation of
the generations line

child
in "child" role

Parents keep the child below the separation of
the generations line in the safety of the child role.
They do this by giving the child the nurturing and
limits that child needs.

Can you recall basking in the safety of the child role?

The appropriate separation is maintained when *parents meet
their child's needs.* It's not enough to put in a good effort. Rather,
it takes meeting the needs of *that* particular child, at *that* stage of
development, in *that* situation—including protecting the child
from challenges and responsibilities that are beyond his or her
capacity to meet.

It is not an easy job. Even in the most loving families, the
needs of children may go wanting. During the losses, changes
and traumas that fate holds for us, even parents who are usually responsive can slide into a permissive or depriving parenting style and not always be able to set aside their own needs to
respond to the child.

Most theorists agree that children need nurturing and limits.

Most psychologists believe that although children *don't* need perfect parenting, they *do* need both sufficient nurturing and protective limits to stay in the child role and thrive. The word *nurturing* usually suggests warmth and loving, while the word *limits* may seem harsh or even frightening. But nurturing and limits are actually two sides of the same coin.

For instance, when I read a story to my son John, tucked into his bed at night, I am nurturing him and it feels *wonderful* to me. The next morning, when I say to him firmly that he must clean up his room *before* he watches cartoons, the experience of setting a limit *does not* feel wonderful. It is serious and hard work. Yet setting that reasonable limit with him is as loving an act as reading to him the night before. Later, after John has stuffed most of the large toys into his closet and his room looks . . . better, he shows me his room and his eyes twinkle with pride—a pride that nurtures his spirit.

Those who champion the needs of children agree on the central role of unconditional positive regard and consistency in healthy child development. Without these, children do not learn to trust their own feelings and honor their own needs.

For instance, Margaret Mahler describes how kids raised without this nurturing and these limits distrust their own feelings. They may be raging with anger that they don't understand and can't express. In fact they may be so confused that they reach for a Popsicle or candy, the most immediate course of comfort.

Marion Woodman, the revered Jungian therapist, confirmed to me during a telephone conversation from her Toronto bungalow that lack of nurturing sows the seeds of emotional overeating. In the absence of emotional sustenance, according to Woodman, food becomes the *physical* substitute for the parental love not experienced by the child. Literally, if they can't get *sweet love*, at least they can get a *sweet*.

Virginia Satir points out that children who are raised without hugs and a welcoming ear begin to feel they don't matter. That sense of being invisible prevents children from seeing themselves. And without a healthy and positive regard for themselves, children have no basis for nurturing themselves. Expecting nothing of themselves, they have no basis for setting limits and developing

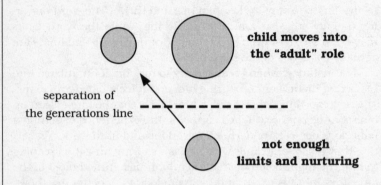

The Child Is in an *Unsafe* Role

child moves into the "adult" role

separation of
the generations line

not enough limits and nurturing

The child does not receive sufficient nurturing
and limits. The child leaves the safety of the child
role and crosses the separation of the
generations line.

At what age did you begin to be in the adult role?

discipline. When life doesn't go well, there are no bootstraps
around with which to pull themselves up.

Alice Miller, whose views on parental narcissism are widely
applauded, observes that lack of nurturing can echo from generation to generation. A child who never experiences a parent's tender love and care becomes an empty well. As adults, searching for
something to fill that void, they turn to external solutions—excess
of eating, drinking, spending, working, fixing or pleasing others.
Never truly filled with emotional sustenance of their own, they
cannot hear the wails of their children over the cry of their own
inner yearnings. What is Miller's conclusion? The emotional
empty cup becomes the legacy of one generation to the next.

Well before the middle of the century, Hilde Bruch pinpointed
many of the dynamics on which *The Diet-Free Solution* is based.
She observed children who were obese and painstakingly docu-

mented their family dynamics. Kids who were overweight tended to have parents that were either too close or too distant to meet their children's needs. Children in overly close, enmeshed families had permissive parents and ended up without separate identities. Without a sense of being an individual, they lost the ability to be sensitive to their own internal signals of hunger and fullness, and tended to overeat.

The child of distant, detached and depriving parents was no better off. When the parents were too removed to know how their children felt, let alone what they needed, nurturing was rare and limits were harsh. These children were emotionally alone and often turned to food to fill their inner abyss.

For those of us with weight problems, there was a critical moment when our needs were put aside for too long, and we did what we had to do—we met *our own* needs. We began to *parent ourselves*.

Unfortunately, there are prices to pay for this violation of the sanctity of childhood. One is chilling isolation. When we as children cross the line into assuming adult roles, we find there is *no* bar mitzvah, *no* coming-of-age party and *no* menstrual marker. We do it *alone*, and we don't even know it is happening. Second, we don't have adult skills, so life doesn't go as well. We miss out on friendships, we are late for school, and we don't know the answer to the math problem. But nobody knows our burden, because we don't dare divulge it. And that is the third price we pay, the tension that comes with faking it. We behave as if to say "I can take care of myself just fine, thank you," when the truth is we can't.

Children are resilient—most grow into accomplished adults.

Despite the inequities and injustices of life, children are resilient. Most grow up and seem to do well in life, becoming good citizens, loyal friends and concerned parents. Yet behind the facade of this accomplished adult life lies an inner turmoil that results from feeling split.

Many people who get training in the method say they feel as if they've always had one foot in adult respectability and the other in sophomoric chaos. The part of them that prematurely rose above the separations of the generation line is now belatedly rel-

The Adult Feels Divided

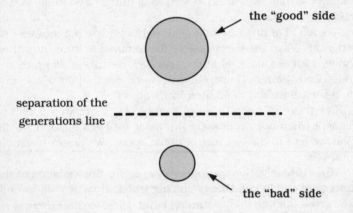

the "good" side

separation of the
generations line

the "bad" side

The child grows up and has many successes. Yet the
part of him or her that didn't get the needed skills in
childhood remains below the line and overeats. The
adult feels divided between the "good" side the world
sees and the "bad" side that overeats.

When did you first feel divided, with a good side and a bad side?

ishing the child role but is also madder than hell, wallowing in
self-pity, making mischief or doing harm.

Katherine, a public defender, told the group with exas-
peration, "I'm asking myself, What is going on? Who am I
really? Am I responsible, strong and energetic, or is the
real truth that I am irresponsible, weak-willed and lazy? I
feel like a Ping-Pong ball, first thinking I'm perfectly OK,
then seeing blatant evidence—in my eating and in my
life—that I'm not."

Paradise is regained. We feel balanced and whole.

As you use the six cures, you begin to feel more authentic and more whole. That sense of being split, confused, all good or all bad, fades away. Feeling whole again does not come from *whipping yourself into shape* or even *taming* the part of you that is *bad*. Rather, it comes from accepting and even feeling compassion for your dark side, your "bad" side, embracing your own mistakes, flaws and flub-ups the way a doting grandmother would.

That acceptance of your "bad" side helps it make the transition into merging with your "good" side so you no longer feel compelled to be either far too good or far too bad. The unconditional love that persuaded the bad side to accept itself is so pervasive that our tendencies to be depressed, hostile, rebellious or self-

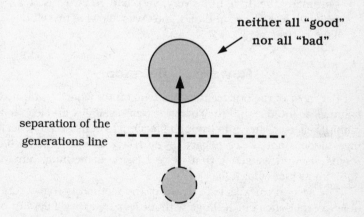

The Adult Feels Whole

neither all "good"
nor all "bad"

separation of the
generations line

As the six cures are mastered, the adult gently
guides the "bad" side above the line with compassion
and self-acceptance. The adult feels whole, and the
overeating subsides.

pitying seem a little silly, and the act of eating the third piece of cake feels abusive rather than nurturing.

Feeling whole knocks the wind out of our appetites.

Katherine's new sense of being whole made her exuberant. "All my rebelliousness and hostility had been coming out in my eating. In a way, I relished eating to excess. It was my way of getting back at everybody. I loved eating handfuls of little chocolate candies at bedtime and stopping off at the convenience store to buy those little packages of powdered sugar doughnuts. Part of me liked being very, very bad and then reforming and being very, very good.

"So I stopped trying to control that part of me. In fact, I began to laugh about it, as if to say, 'Gee, that hostile, rebellious part of me wants doughnuts again. Oh, dear, when is she going to stop doing that anyway? Maybe never!' Somehow just accepting these tendencies in myself rather than trying to fix them was a way of giving them love and respect. Miraculously, that attitude of compassion made the drive to be very, very bad go away. Now I really do feel whole, and all it took was allowing myself to be imperfect."

Reward 2. Balance

For most of us, our feelings are *way* out of whack, *far* out of balance, so intense that they override our sensibility and lead to a painful roller-coaster ride through life. Others of us keep our feelings hidden, and we're nagged by our lack of spontaneity; life seems dry and we sense that we're missing something, but we don't know just what it is.

The second unexpected reward of the method is that we are able to experience our feelings without fear that they'll get out of control. We can maintain our inner balance.

Jack either rode an emotional roller coaster or was just plain numb. There was no in between.

Jack, an attorney who specialized in intellectual properties, shared a law practice with three buddies from his grammar school days. He was married to his former secretary, and seemed genuinely optimistic, but he never really opened up to anyone about his feelings and thoughts. In our training meetings, he shared a side of himself that few people saw.

"No one would know it but I have three moods: high, low and off. I turn off my feelings most of the time during my work day out of expediency. I just want to focus on getting the job done. At social occasions, there's lots of eating, drinking and small talk, so I'm on a kind of unreal high. At night the lows hit, but my wife, Gina, knows to leave me alone then, and never presses me about my eating or drinking. What I don't like is that either my moods are extreme or I have no feelings at all."

Jack's three moods reflected how out of emotional balance he was, which contributed to his weight problem.

Unbalanced feelings: highs, lows and numbness

These unbalanced moods arise when the pure feelings of joy or anger or love or sadness have been distorted by weak nurturing or ineffective limits. For example, the pure feelings that arise when receiving a warm hug from someone who loves us may be happiness or contentment. But if the experience is filtered through harsh, judgmental thinking—"I don't deserve this" or "They probably aren't sincere"—we might feel panic or depression instead. Or the feelings the hug arouses in us may be so intense that we can't handle them and turn cold and numb to stop feeling anything.

Balanced feelings: earned rewards and essential pain

Earned rewards are the normal positive moods that come from the good things in life: feeling proud when we clinch a deal, joyful when we find strawberries on sale, content when we are in the company of a trusted friend. Rewarded by these good feelings, we're inclined to repeat the behaviors that produced them.

Essential pain is the discomfort we experience when things don't go well: angry but not hostile when we're criticized, sad but not depressed when there are disappointments and afraid but not

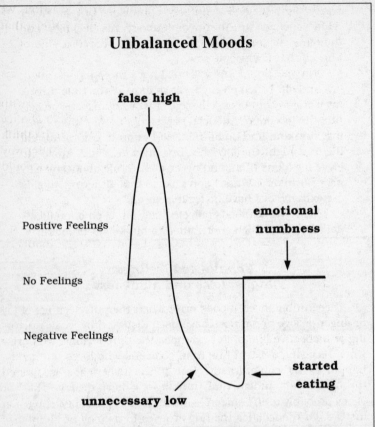

Unbalanced Moods

false high

emotional numbness

Positive Feelings

No Feelings

Negative Feelings

started eating

unnecessary low

Without the six cures, we are prone to false highs, unnecessary lows and numbness. We don't experience the normal ups and downs that prompt us to change and grow.

panicked in the face of danger. Oddly enough, the pure feelings of anger, sadness, fear and guilt are not that painful.

In fact, the sadness that comes with any disappointment can be faced immediately, it doesn't pile up, and soon the feeling begins to fade. We take a deep breath, feel as awful as we must feel, then watch the feeling fade and learn from our experience.

We go on with the business of making our lives even better. We learn from that pain and are less likely to repeat a pattern that hasn't been rewarding for us.

How do balanced moods benefit us?

Earned rewards and essential pain prod us in two ways—with rewards and punishments. As a result we wake up and change our behavior by saying to ourselves either, "That felt good, I think I'll do that again," or, conversely, "That hurts, I'll find a better way next time." As we do so, we change, grow and prosper. Jack could see this in himself.

"When I eat and drink too much at night, I'm not in emotional balance. I don't feel sad about it the next morning. Instead I either feel numb—I just don't think about

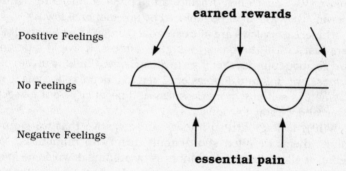

Balanced Moods

Positive Feelings

earned rewards

No Feelings

Negative Feelings

essential pain

The normal ups and down of life benefit us. We experience feelings and learn from them. We continue doing things that reward us and seek alternatives to those that cause us pain.

it—or, if I've been on a real bender of eating or drinking, the next morning I am hard on myself.

"I say, 'Why don't you wise up? What's wrong with you anyway?' and get so depressed and so caught up in how revolting I am that I completely miss feeling the sadness of the situation. My attention is no longer on the situation; it's on feeling sorry for myself and feeling depressed about my lack of control. I don't change. I just get stuck in the groove and keep the pattern going year after year."

Jack was right. If he had truly felt his pure sadness about being alone and his pure disappointment about his lack of physical vitality, he probably wouldn't have continued to be so isolated, and might have overeaten and overdrunk less. However, Jack didn't feel those feelings, because they were blocked by his unbalanced moods.

The seductiveness of unbalanced moods

False highs feel good just the way earned rewards do, but they differ in one respect: *they aren't real.* Based on inherently unstable distortion in our thinking, false highs are both chaotic and elusive. We sense their fragility and clutch them more tightly, knowing they will soon be replaced by an emotional low.

Unnecessary lows are like essential pain, but last longer. If we were just to feel the basic feeling of sadness, it would fade and we'd go about our day. Yet if we invite negative thinking to join our sadness, we sink into depression. Then that depression calls to its playmates—self-pity, powerlessness and negativity—our low gets lower, and we stay low longer.

When feelings are so intense and negative that we cannot handle them, we often short-circuit them with numbness. Not feeling at all. We bring on numbness by stuffing down some food, turning on the tube or concentrating on pleasing others. Although numbness is a welcome escape, like false highs and unnecessary lows it keeps us from experiencing the balanced feelings necessary for improving our lives.

Which moods are most common for you?

These unbalanced feelings can be harmful, not just because they hurt or because we overeat in response to them. The biggest

Common Feelings in the Five Moods

False highs

rebellious arrogant greedy elated manic
fantasizing stuffed all-powerful impervious

Earned rewards

grateful happy secure proud rested
pleased safe satisfied loved healthy

Numbness
no feelings

Essential pain

angry sad afraid guilty disappointed
tired vulnerable hungry lonely sick

Unnecessary Lows
hostile depressed panic abandoned
self-pitying powerless exhausted stuffed
ashamed

harm they do is to keep us from growing. We become so involved in our low that we completely miss the essential pain of the situation.

For instance, your mother calls and says something decidedly nasty to you. It isn't the first time. If you allow yourself to feel your balanced feelings—anger, sadness and fear, for instance—you might develop a way of handling her next phone call differently. Perhaps you'll tell her how the criticism feels or decide to keep phone calls brief.

If negative, powerless thoughts surface instead, you might say to yourself, "I will always have to take disrespect from her.

She's a terrible person." Those negative, powerless thoughts transform your anger into hostility, and your sadness becomes depression. You are in an unnecessary low and feel immobilized. In fact you feel so distressed that you completely bypass the essential pain involved.

The essential pain is that listening to your mother being nasty feels bad. To stop her will require you to back away or confront her. If you back away or confront her, she may reject you. Feeling that essential pain stimulates and empowers you to respond to that reality and make coherent decisions about what to do.

If instead you allow your inner voice to move your anger to hostility and your sadness to depression, finding ways to solve the problem won't even cross your mind. You'll be too wrapped up in how *awful* you feel. What you really need in order to grow and change—that is, to solve problems and take action—will not occur. The next time your mother calls you will tolerate her nasty comments and again end up feeling hostile and depressed. You will not change, and neither will your life.

The false highs and unnecessary lows of dieting

An example of an intoxicating false high is the one Jack experienced when he was dieting. Jack had been on two physician-supervised fasts, and in each instance he enjoyed every second of being in complete control of his eating. He was on cloud nine.

Moreover, in the back of his mind were visions of how things would be when the diet was over—he would have the perfect body, the perfect life and never again would his evenings be lost to excessive food and drink. But Jack was headed for emotional disaster.

During each diet, Jack sank into an unnecessary low when, at some critical point, the false high had run its course. No longer was he buoyed up with the expectation that his diet would be easy and the anticipation of fabulous results. What's more, his negative, powerless thoughts hastened his plunge into an unnecessary low. Rather than rebounding from that emotional low, he stayed in it, wallowing in large doses of both self-pity and depression until another false high, a further unnecessary low or the lure of emotional numbness overtook him.

Using the six cures puts our emotional life back in balance.

As Jack mastered the cures, he became adept at turning unbalanced moods into balanced ones as readily as a spatula turns over a pancake on the grill. Consider how Jack used the six cures to bring him back into emotional balance.

"This diet is never going to work. I've had it. I'm going to eat pizza and drink beer tonight for dinner. I'm going to take every naked chicken breast and every stalk of broccoli in the house and dump it in the garbage. Enough is enough!"

Jack pauses and goes inside himself to use the six cures. He begins by checking his feelings and needs, asking himself the questions involved in strong nurturing:

"How do I feel?"

Depressed. Sick of dieting. Angry that it is so hard. Angry that I have to even deal with food and weight. I hate it.

"What do I need?"

I need to be easier on myself. I'm pushing myself to eat too little and be too "good."

"Do I need to ask for help?"

No, this is permission I can give myself.

Next Jack makes sure that negative, powerless thoughts aren't sending him into emotional imbalance, by asking himself the questions of the effective limits cure:

"What do I expect?"

To lose three pounds this week. To feel and look very different right away. To be able to deny myself food.

"Is that reasonable?

No.

"What is reasonable?"

That I lose about a pound per week, eat a little healthier and take several months to show a big difference.

"Are my thoughts powerful and positive?"

No.

"What could I say to myself that would be?"

That I'm doing the best I can, that I will make my goal in time and I don't have to be perfect to be wonderful.

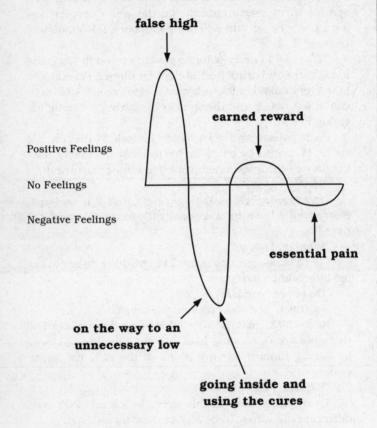

The Cures Return Us to Emotional Balance

false high

earned reward

Positive Feelings

No Feelings

Negative Feelings

essential pain

**on the way to an
unnecessary low**

**going inside and
using the cures**

Using the cures returns us to inner balance. We
experience the balanced feelings that help us
grow and change.

"What is the essential pain?"
    That this isn't easy. That it takes time and that it won't
change everything about me, just my weight.

"What feeling does that bring up for you?"
Sadness, fear.
"Can you allow yourself just to feel the feelings of sadness and fear, knowing that within a few moments they will fade?"
Yes, I think so. . . .*(Sigh)* That's better. It's gone. I think I can go on with eating healthily now.

Back in emotional balance, Jack's pizza and beer aren't so important.

Finally, Jack makes any needed adjustments in body and lifestyle by touching on the remaining cures.
"Are my body and lifestyle in balance?"
Yes, except that I need to get some exercise this evening. I think I'll stop at the gym on my way home from work.

The entire process took only a few minutes, but it put Jack back in control of his inner balance and supported him in following through with eating healthfully. That evening, instead of launching into eating and drinking, he went to the gym and had a light supper.

Reward 3. Sanctuary

The third unexpected reward of mastering the method is sanctuary. Instead of being afraid of your inner life, you have the security of knowing that at any time, no matter how difficult things become, you can go inside yourself and find safety in your own personal sanctuary.

Nichole, a 33-year-old artist and mother of three, was relieved to discover that as she mastered the cures and lost the extra sixteen pounds she'd carried around since the birth of her last child, she acquired a sense of sanctuary.

She reflected, "I am the motherly, loving type, but the voice inside me was not always loving. It was a bizarre combination of my parents' voices: my mother's, who was the first to notice what was wrong with me—my missed piano note or my turned-up collar—and my dad's, with its negative and unhappy expectations.

"By the time I was an adult, the voice inside me was anything but safe. But no more. Even when my art submissions are turned down and the kids are jumping out of their skin being cooped up inside on a rainy day, I can take a deep breath and turn my awareness to my inner life. What I find there is a fairly accepting, supportive voice. It feels great!"

Reward 4. Intimacy

Intimacy is luscious, the emotional equivalent of swirling a chocolate truffle on the tongue. It comes in many different forms: a baby's closeness with its mother, teamwork with friends on the ball field, laughing at Dad's corny jokes. It might be the comfortable intimacy of a soul mate or an unexpected electric moment with a new friend. Whatever the source, most of us have had some tastes of the sweet succor of intimacy, and learned how it uplifts the soul and warms the heart.

Sex? Yes. Intimacy? Let me think about it . . .

Although intimacy can be uplifting and warming, it can also be absolutely *terrifying*. Our hearts, our souls and, at times, our bodies are exposed and vulnerable. We take the risk that the person we love and trust may, when we least expect it, magnify our every blemish and flat out reject us. And sometimes we may unwittingly surrender to the compelling will of another. Intimacy is an adult activity—because of the risks.

Fortunately, the risks of intimacy can be lessened by effective boundaries, a kind of psychological membrane that lets in the good and keeps out the bad. But to be effective in providing us with safety and closeness in relationships, a boundary must be neither too thick nor too thin. Conveniently, nurturing and limits make thin boundaries thicker and slim down thick ones so that the possibility of intimacy is enhanced.

The safety of boundaries that are neither too thick nor too thin . . .

A boundary that is too thin will leave us with no sense of our own separateness. When we don't know or can't identify our own feelings and needs, expressing them is virtually impossible. We risk being taken over by others, swept away by the power of their feelings and needs. Furthermore, if a relationship ends, we do not possess the separate sense of ourselves needed to pick up the pieces and go on. When our boundaries are too thin, we are rarely capable of allowing ourselves to be seen for who we truly are. We aren't clear who we are, and we may have revealed to our partners only the person we think they want us to be.

Too thin for her own good

Deirdre, a robust Canadian woman who was the adored office manager for a group of orthodontists, shared with me, "Oh, there's no question that I'm the one with the skinny boundaries. I form two kinds of relationships. One is with my women friends who have skinny boundaries too, and we soak in each other's feelings. I have to catch myself or I'll start minding their business instead of my own and then getting mad at them when they don't do it my way.

"The other kind of relationship is the kind I have with my boss and also my husband. They both have boundaries as thick as leather. But I like it because it makes me feel safer, because their relationships with me force me to have thicker boundaries myself. It's as if I borrow some of their boundary from them.

"The only problem is that I wish they were both more open. The more closed they get, the more I pound on the door and want them to respond to me. It's taken me a long time to realize that the harder I pound on the door, the longer it will take them to come out. I used to think it was their problem, but I have grown to see it as mine, too. It's not safe for my boss, or my husband either, to be close to me if my own boundary is so skinny and fragile."

On the other hand, a big thick boundary allows us *only* a sense of our separateness. We're so self-aware, it's difficult to feel the feelings of others and to develop empathy and compassion. Without those connecting emotions, we have no reason to meet the needs of others and we risk falling into emotional isolation.

Moreover, when our boundaries are too thick, our inherent goodness is not apparent to others. They don't get to know us well enough to care about us, and as a result, we may neither give nor get the love we need.

So thick that he walled himself away

Ron, a man of tremendous energy, was typical of someone with thicker boundaries. Manager of a computer software company, he lived alone and was always on the run.

"I can't say relationships are the focal point of my life, because I have many interests that gratify me—my computer work, my investments, kayaking and a collection of antique engines. My relationships haven't been particularly close. I've had friends at work, and I was married for four years, but now I've been single for six years.

"I'm sure I could get more satisfaction in my romantic life if my boundaries weren't so thick, but most of the women who are attracted to me are kind of hysterical. They seem to want to own me, rather than just to enjoy my company. I know some of their neediness comes from reacting to my aloofness, but their frenzy doesn't make it any easier for me to be close to them. I also don't want that closeness, because it inevitably results in breaking up. I am a very critical, exacting person, and some of that rubs off onto the people I get close to.

"My boundaries definitely need to get thinner, but for me the first step is to become more skilled at nurturing and limits so that my inner voice is kinder."

Using the six cures makes thick boundaries a little thinner . . .

Every time those of us with *thick* boundaries use the strong nurturing cure and express our feelings and needs, we open up a little bit more. Moreover, each time we use the effective limits cure, our inner life becomes more positive and less judgmental, so we don't fear being seen for who we are. All of this chips away— just a little—at the extra distance our thick boundary has put between us and intimate relationships. In time, we notice that our relationships hold more warmth, and this closeness feels safer to us than it has ever felt before. Intimacy, the most potent appetite suppressant, can now walk in.

Intimacy Self–Test
Assessing Your Boundaries

Check the characteristics that are true for you?

Thick Boundaries
____ I keep my feelings to myself.

____ I'm not a talker.

____ I don't really want to hear other people's problems.

____ I keep my distance from other people's feelings.

Thin Boundaries
____ I tell my feelings to almost anyone who will listen.

____ I am a talker.

____ I enjoy listening to other people's problems.

____ I get caught up in the feelings of others.

My boundaries tend to be:

too thick   **too thin**

sometimes thick/sometimes thin

. . . and thin ones just a little thicker.

Quite the opposite is true for those of us with skinny boundaries. Each time we use the strong nurturing cure, we define our own individual feelings and needs, which gives us the distance and detachment we need to be close to others without losing ourselves. Likewise, each time we use the effective limits cure we enhance the strength of our self-definition. To master the cure, we must face our own expectations and thoughts and be willing to accept life's inevitable discomfort. Each time we do, we strengthen the membrane between ourselves and the rest of the world. Together these cures bolster our boundaries just enough to allow for healthy intimacy.

Paul and Angie were a good example of a couple who possessed more than enough luck and compatibility for a good relationship but lacked the boundaries to make intimacy safe and attainable. Paul's boundaries were too thick, and Angie's were too thin.

Angie enrolled in a Solution group at the university. Paul came to the orientation, but he decided to master the method on his own. As Angie and Paul solved their weight problems through the six cures, their relationship developed a new level of intimacy and trust.

Angie began to contain her feelings more and soothe herself. She stopped running to Paul with every hurt or need because increasingly she had the capacity to follow through and meet her own needs.

Paul felt less threatened by Angie's emotional neediness and psychological intrusiveness, so he could more easily relax with Angie and open up to her. If he shared something personal with her, he could trust that she wouldn't become overly anxious or driven to rescue him from it. They now rarely play out their old pattern of Angie crowding Paul and Paul distancing from her. They found a balance between them that was safe and sparked by intimacy.

Reward 5. Vibrancy

Richard told me that his weight never really bothered him except that he felt so lethargic. In fact, he said he only tried the method because he was approaching his fiftieth birthday and felt life was passing him by. He wanted to fulfill his dream of being fit again, which was, according to him, to be "like an iron man."

At our initial meeting, Richard said, "I was a jock in high school and ate like a horse. I'd come home from football practice after school and down half a box of raisin bran and a quart of milk. I remember that feeling of being slightly sore all over with my muscles still hot from exercising. In those days, I felt like I had the world by the tail, and right now in my life I want that feeling back."

Richard got that feeling back, but it took more than just going after physical fitness with a vengeance. Within a month of starting out, he had already injured himself by pulling a back muscle. This had happened before and was always followed by a month of pain and six months of depression and inactivity.

This time was different. Richard ratcheted down his expectations a few notches and kept up lower body exercise during the month of pain. He expressed a lot of feelings—utter frustration, poignant fear and a fair amount of fury—and began increasing his exercise slowly and steadily.

By the end of his training session, Richard felt great. "I've never before been able to stick with exercise in the long run. Effective limits gave me more staying power than I've ever had. My endorphins are pumping away, so most nights I feel upbeat and relaxed. I think people really underrate how much being completely fit changes your entire life."

Vivian was not a jock like Richard and she had never been fit before in her entire adult life. Yet vibrancy meant more to her than the twenty-one pounds she lost by using the method.

"I never liked to exercise. Part of it was that I don't like to perspire and I'm not very athletic, but I think it was more emotional than anything. Exercise would bring up feelings about my body being wrong and the way my brother would ridicule my breasts when I was developing. So gaining some body pride and being able to express some of those past hurts really freed me up to move my body freely.

"Now I'm really, really fit and I love it, mainly because it gives me a sense of power—and even grace. I move better, and that makes me enjoy everything more. I just scheduled a whitewater rafting trip for this summer.

Things like that I would never even have considered doing before."

It was fabulous to watch Richard and Vivian become so vibrant. They exuded not only physical vitality but optimism and powerfulness. They now looked like people who loved life and weren't afraid to grab hold and run with it.

Reward 6. Spirituality

I first began to understand the role of spirituality in the six cures many years ago when I was working at the university with overweight teens and their parents.

It was the parents who were having difficulty witnessing their teens' pain about weight: the clothes that wouldn't fit, the phone that didn't ring and the teams their children couldn't make. In the midst of their frustration, many parents drifted away from setting reasonable limits with their teens and entered the arena of over-control.

One particular fall evening, the discussion in the parents' meeting centered on how to force their teens to toe the line with a depriving diet and a rigorous exercise schedule. One parent said, "I just can't let go. I can't let Kirk be self-destructive. He's ruining his body; his chest is bigger than mine now and he even has stretch marks. It breaks my heart to see him ruining his life."

The other parents promptly agreed that setting limits took accepting the essential pain that they could not control their adolescents' behavior. The issue at hand seemed so clear that I asked the inevitable question: "What would happen if you did let go? What can you trust that gives you some assurance that things will work out? What safety net, benevolent force or basic strength do you believe in?"

In this group, they all agreed that they didn't believe they could let go, because there was nothing they could trust to make things work out. Of course I was surprised, but not for long.

That evening, I called Velia Frost, the family therapist involved with the university's Solution group for children and families, which is called the Shapedown Program. Her response was to the point: "Why would these parents think there was a safety net or a spiritual being in the world? Many of these parents weren't nurtured well growing up. They had no experience of any kind of safety net or beneficial force. Why should they have trust that it will be there for their children?"

Velia's point spotlighted the potential for the method to result in spiritual changes. People who let go of external solutions and reconnect with what is good within them could certainly become more spiritually aware and influenced. First of all, external solutions effectively block a spirituality that is within us ready to be developed. Second, there may be an innate hungering for the spiritual, which takes over as the inner life develops. A prophet once said, "Every man has a God-shaped hole in his heart." Enriching the inner life may naturally result in filling that void.

In fact, the spiritual deepening that might arise through using these tools could ultimately be the power of the program. Nothing so quickly catalyzes a personal transformation as a spiritual awakening. As it happens, the follow-up research on the method has surprised even me. Two years after beginning to use the method, participants who reported a spiritual deepening lost on the average *five times as much* weight as those who did not report a spiritual change.

When these participants were interviewed, it was clear that the spiritual shifts came over time and emerged in subtle ways. Some participants said they used their religion's practices more frequently. Others felt a greater presence of the divine in their lives, and still others said they had a heightened appreciation for the mystery and grace of life.

Putting it all together . . .

The elegance of the design of weight problems turns out to be stunning. In all the medical literature the most intractable, stubborn and frustrating of the common problems is being overweight. Sure, people take their medicines like they should, switch from butter to olive oil and cut down on smoking. But in recent years a scant few of us have resolved our weight issues. The sheer frustration of it turns out to be part of why solving weight problems rewards us so much. If solving a weight problem were as easy as buying canola oil instead of butter and taking pills on time every day, the rewards of it would probably be small.

Instead, weight problems are such difficult nuts to crack that we must go far deeper inside if we are to achieve the success we desire. As it turns out, there is no easy way out of a weight prob-

The Solution

We master the Six Cures.
1. Strong Nurturing
2. Effective Limits
3. Body Pride
4. Good Health
5. Balanced Eating
6. Mastery Living

↓

The agony ends.

We recieve the Six Rewards.

1. Chaos	1. Integration
2. Imbalance	2. Balance
3. Peril	3. Sanctuary
4. Isolation	4. Intimacy
5. Lethargy	5. Vibrancy
6. Emptiness	6. Spirituality

↓

**The weight problem is solved.
Our life is transformed.**

lem. We can either live with it, numbing ourselves to the pain, or rely on one external solution after another: first fasts, then packaged meals, then drugs. Or we can possess the courage and skills to step into the ring with the *true* causes of weight problems—and make peace with them.

And the elegance of the design is that by making peace with our weight problem, we overcome the consequences of an unresponsive early environment and bring ourselves life's richest rewards:

- A sense of integration replaces feelings of chaos.

- Moods become balanced rather than high, low or numb.

- A sense of sanctuary replaces feelings of peril.

- Intimacy is enhanced and isolation lessens.

- Lethargy gives way to personal vibrancy.

- Emptiness fades and a sense of the spiritual deepens.

Moreover, there is a legacy of our experience of chaos, imbalance, peril, isolation, lethargy and emptiness. These are the most common human discomforts, and because we have been there and back, we can empathize with the discomforts of others in a far deeper way than we could if we were raised in a "perfect" environment with "perfect" parents. And because we are aware of the pain of life, we awaken to its supreme pleasures as well. Experiencing and resolving our weight problem has enabled us to be far more human and far more alive than we would have been if life had been "perfect."

The next step is a personal one . . .

The next step in your weight solution is to personalize it. That's right. No matter how universal the cures, how you approach your weight issue has to do with individual matters. In the next part of this book you will look inward at the true causes of your weight issue and determine for yourself whether or not your weight really matters.

Part 2
Your Personal Solution

*Looking more closely at yourself:
your patterns, your risks, your desires.*

Your Own Solution Inventory

In this chapter, you will complete your own Solution Inventory, which will customize the method to your individual needs. Chances are, all the causes are important to you, but some have influenced your weight more than others. This chapter presents an opportunity for you to fine-tune your solution and focus on the cures that will be most beneficial to you.

You will also find answers to some of the most common questions about weight: are weight problems in my genes? and what are the roots of my tendency to gain weight? And I'll give you a close look at one person's experience responding to these questions.

Stanley, a family doctor at San Francisco General Hospital, whose sister, Kristin, had attended a talk I'd given the previous month in St. Louis, called me about the method. Kristin had begun to lose weight, called Stanley and told him about the method, and he was inquiring about it for his patients as well as for himself.

What are the real causes of my weight?

- What is the role of genetics in my body size?
- Is my pattern depriving, permissive or both?
- What is my personal profile of the six cures?

You see, Stanley and Kristin had both experienced weight problems since childhood. As kids, they had shared forbidden foods, foods like cellophane-wrapped packages of chocolate cupcakes with squiggles on top and pans of Sara Lee frozen brownies—only partially thawed.

As adults their mutual weight problems had become a source of emotional "glue" between them. Stanley had convinced Kristin to cancel her marriage plans in part because her fiancé had pressured her to lose weight. And when Stanley had gained thirty pounds during his residency, Kristin had shipped him a crate of Florida grapefruit.

The timing of Kristin's call to Stanley about *The Diet-Free Solution* couldn't have been better for his weight, which had always been a barometer of his stress and had gone up in the past year. Stanley's stress level was perfectly understandable. He had taken on, in addition to a full load of patient care, an AIDS research project that was aimed at finding ways to prevent the disease in inner-city adolescents. Although Stanley loved the work and got a certain "high" from the frenzied pace it required, he wasn't happy about his increasing weight. When we spoke, he had many questions, including the following.

"My family is heavy. Is it in my genes?"

You may have a sibling, parents and even a grandparent who are also heavy and wonder if you're fighting a losing battle with weight. You might even ask yourself, Is it my genetic destiny to be on the rounder, fluffier or bigger side? Stanley was no different. His sister and parents were also heavy, and he wondered if it was just his genetic destiny to be big.

We all know people with "round genes," the kind that encourage the body to vacuum up every trace of energy consumed and deposit it in just the place they'd *least* like to have it. If you've read the obesity headlines of the newspapers in the last few years—which suggest that obesity is all in the genes—you may have been inclined to throw in the towel, deciding that your weight is as static as your eye color.

How much weight do genes carry?

Although the media portray the genetic influence on weight as a guarantee of perpetual weight problems, science says differently. The influence of genetic factors varies from individual to individual, and researchers who study such factors—Claude Bouchard, F. Xavier Pi-Sunyer and Albert J. Stunkard—conclude that *at most* 5 to 25 percent of one's weight can be attributed solely to genetics.

What seems to be important is not the extent to which one's genes invite the number on the scale to increase, but how they interact with one's lifestyle. Due to their genetic makeup, some people exhibit a greater tendency to gain weight, or more *elasticity*, than others.

For instance, the Pima Indians—who have unique genes that are highly elastic—can eat even small amounts of extra food and gain weight. On the other hand, many people with "skinny genes" can binge eat, habitually indulge or watch television for days on end, and there is no effect on their weight.

There are considerable data that support the view that one's genetics is not the whole story. Stanley Garn from the University of Michigan reviewed a broad spectrum that followed people over several decades. He found that body weight varies *tremendously* over time. In fact, according to one study by Dr. Garn, 40 percent of women and 60 percent of men who were initially obese were normal weight two decades later. Based on these data, it is clear that weight is not immutable.

If being overweight is primarily genetic, how could it increase 31 percent nationally in ten years?

Recent research has suggested that Garn is right. Weight—for most of us—is quite open to change.

That evidence is based on nationally representative samples of Americans surveyed with the National Health and Nutrition Examination Survey (NHANES). According to the results of this survey, the prevalence of obesity has shown a phenomenal upward trend in the last two decades. In adults, obesity rates recently have jumped 31 percent—from 24.5 percent in 1976–1980 to a full 33.3 percent in 1988–1991. What's more, we have seen a similar trend in children, with child obesity skyrocketing 54 percent in the last two decades and adolescent obesity up a full 39 percent.

Indeed, steep inclines in obesity compel us to look at lifestyle factors—not genetic predestination—as a primary cause. But what aspect of lifestyle is fueling this dramatic weight gain among Americans? People who quit smoking gain weight, and smoking rates have plummeted in the last decade, so perhaps reduced smoking is the culprit. Alternatively, demographers might argue that overweight women have higher fertility rates, thus possibly increasing the presence of genetic obesity in the national gene pool. Perhaps it's all those hours at the computer, television and video. The best estimate is that these causes have minor effects on the increase in obesity rates.

The evidence points to what we eat. Despite the no-fat hype in the marketplace and the proliferation of such products as fat-free brownies, sugar-free and fat-free ice cream, and no-fat chips, we are eating *more* fat and *more* calories now than in 1978.

How could this be? Everyone we know is conscious of fat grams.

Diets in 1990 were lower in fat as a percentage of calories; the total amount of fat we consumed actually *increased*. Fat intake rose from an average of 709 calories per day in 1978 to 748 calories per day in 1990, up 6 percent despite a flood of information about the dangers of obesity and the elevated risk of developing heart disease and cancer from high-fat diets. It wasn't just fat in diets that increased in the last decade. The average number of total calories consumed exploded during this period, rising to 2,200, up a startling 12 percent from 1969.

Body changes brought on by weight can make you gain more weight.

Research shows that although both lifestyle and genetics may play a role in adding weight to our frames, in most cases, lifestyle is more influential. However, regardless of whether a weight gain was caused by round genes or too many pizzas, *that extra body fat soon takes on a life of its own.*

Unfair as it is, the fatter we are, the fatter we are apt to become. It's almost as if Mother Nature were saying, "There you have it. Either do something major about your weight problem or I'll make it worse and worse!"

Luckily, there are some strategies that can help offset these biological drives toward weight gain—or at least slow them down. Seven biological factors are understood to contribute to weight gain. These range from having a slower metabolic rate to having more lipoprotein lipase, an enzyme that transports fat from the blood into the cells. In addition, there are variations among people in thermogenesis. Thermogenesis is the ability to transform calories from the Thanksgiving feast, the late-night binge or the restaurant excess into heat. That heat escapes the body, rather than becoming stored on the body.

Moreover, if we gained weight at various vulnerable points in our lives, in the early years, in puberty or during pregnancy, we probably have fat cells that won't shrink below a certain size. These fat cells are what is called *biologically refractory,* meaning that the size at which they are comfortable is bigger than a size that would keep us lean. If we lose too much weight, our fat cells may throw their weight around—literally—and send the needle on the scale up again.

The importance of insulin . . .

Insulin is one of the body hormones that regulates how the food we eat is metabolized. Insulin helps the glucose in our blood enter our cells and promotes the conversion of blood sugar into fat and the storage of that fat in fat cells. The more overweight we are, particularly when we carry fat on the abdomen, the less our cells respond to insulin.

Why? Because there are fewer "doors" on each cell where insulin can work, and those doors are less open than when we were leaner. This phenomenon is called *insulin resistance.* If a cell doesn't respond to insulin, our body makes more insulin and shoots it into the blood, attempting to open the glucose doors. In fact, the heavier we are and the more we overeat, the more insulin we produce.

Having too much insulin in the blood is called *hyperinsuline-mia.* This condition affects one in four adults. Recent studies suggest that if you are overweight and your body makes more insulin as a result, the insulin levels in your brain do something rather peculiar. They fall proportionally. That change in the brain level of insulin seems to have an effect on the appetite. Our natural brakes on eating become blunted, and our body continues to *think* it needs food even when it *doesn't*. So we eat more and gain weight.

Furthermore, having proportionally less insulin in the brain appears to cause the body to burn up less fat as well. We hold on to more body fat, and our weight continues to mount.

The good news is that with weight loss, this insulin resistance and its effect on promoting weight gain diminish and may disappear completely! Meanwhile, even before you lose weight, the skills of Balanced Eating and Mastering Living can help minimize the weight-gaining effects of insulin resistance.

"How would I know if these factors affected me?"

The question is really twofold: One, do you have genes that make your body apt to gain weight? And two, do you have certain other body factors that fuel weight gain regardless of genetics?

Let's begin with the question about genetics. The availability of genetic testing for obesity is a long way off, and when it comes, there won't be one test but many, because at nearly every leg of the journey from thin to fat, genes play a role. In fact, there is mounting evidence that metabolic rate, hunger and fullness signals and perhaps even spontaneous activity can be inherited.

However, we can still estimate our risk for having round genes by noticing certain of our characteristics. Several characteristics have been associated with genetic obesity. So by taking the test below, you'll see if having round genes affects your weight.

Stanley was overweight by the age of 5. Studies have shown that the child with a genetic propensity to gain weight will begin adding body fat at that time; those with skinnier genes tend to wait until later to add a soft layer of fat under their skin.

There are other earmarks of being genetically overweight—having obese parents, little sensitivity to signals of hunger and satisfaction and keeping weight on despite healthy lifestyles. Stanley had none of these characteristics, so he had a score of 2, which suggested that genes might have a moderate influence on his weight.

Is it my genes?

Please check the characteristics below that
are true for you.

_____ overweight at ages 5 to 7

_____ one parent was overweight

_____ the other parent was also overweight

_____ can't sense hunger and fullness

_____ stay overweight even when habits are healthy

Scoring

Score 1 point for each of the characteristics
you checked.

How likely it is that your genes contribute to
your weight?

0	1	2	3	4 or 5
very low	**low**	**moderate**	**high**	**very high**

What about the other
body factors?

If you scored high on the genetic test, then body factors are
probably adding to your weight. However, even if you didn't gain
weight because of genetics, if you carry it in the middle or high on
your body, many of these same body factors may be at work.
Fortunately, there are many effective strategies for counteracting
these influences, which I will show you.

You might also want to ask your physician for some additional
tests, the most important of which is a *fasting glucose test* to
screen for diabetes. Unfortunately, there is no test for insulin

resistance, but if you carry weight in the middle or high on your body, you very likely are affected by it.

In addition, if you think your metabolic rate is abnormally low, you can always inquire about getting a thyroid function test, but typically it is unnecessary. Weight gain caused by thyroid disease is mild, and the disease itself has many other clinical signs your physician can point out to you, such as cold hands and feet, a coarsening of the facial features, hair loss and constipation.

Unless your tests showed an abnormal thyroid function, you wouldn't be advised to take thyroid medication. Not only are there potential side effects, but about 75 percent of any weight you lost from taking them would be lean tissue rather than fat. Of course, that's counterproductive to a weight solution. You want to maintain as much energy-burning lean tissue as possible so as to maximize your caloric needs and prevent weight gain. Compared to the near comatose levels of energy required by body fat, muscle tissue does handstands to increase your caloric needs.

> Stanley was reluctant to have any tests done. He knew his metabolism was on the slow side. He isn't the sort of person who fidgets or can't sit still, but he didn't have any signs of a thyroid problem. He told me that he was probably insulin resistant because his mother was at his age and he had a classic apple-shaped body.
>
> After some hesitancy, he had a fasting glucose test and it turned out that he had diabetes, which both scared him and encouraged him to do something about his weight.

So now we know. What can we *do* about it?

Many of the body causes of weight gain can be counterbalanced to some extent through the six cures. I'll show you some subtle adjustments you can make within the six cures to enhance this effect.

> Once Stanley knew for certain that he had diabetes, the kind that is mainly caused by weight problems and doesn't usually require insulin, he was motivated to take off his weight. As a physician, he knew full well that losing

The Body Factors That Affect Weight

The body factor . . .   The cures to use . . .

1. A slower metabolism.

You may have a slower metabolism (the calories needed to fuel basic body functions). This accounts for 60 to 70 percent of energy needs; thus even a small decrease can affect your weight.

Mastery Living

Increase your strength training so you have more of the muscle that burns calories; increase the intensity of your exercise to raise your metabolic rate.

2. A tendency to move less.

You may have a tendency to move less. Less energy is expended and further weight gain is more likely.

Effective Limits and Mastery Living

Face the essential pain that you must be physically active in order to solve your weight problem. Find forms of exercise you enjoy. Also, use effective limits to follow through in exercising 30 to 90 minutes per day.

The body factor . . .	The cures to use . . .
3. More likely to store the fat you eat as body fat. You may have higher levels of lipoprotein lipase, the enzyme that deposits fat. It is unclear whether this is due to genetics or a result of other factors, including being female, or overeating. This level stays high even after weight loss.	**Effective Limits and Balanced Eating** Face the essential pain that solving your weight problem may require a very low-fat pattern of eating. Focus on eating more of the light foods you find satisfying and delicious.
4. Reduced loss of calories after overeating. You may be more apt to gain weight after overeating because of blunted thermogenesis (fewer calories lost as body heat after eating).	**Strong Nurturing and Balanced Eating** Master Strong Nurturing so food pleasure is less important. Use Balanced Eating to stop eating when you are just satisfied, not full. Appreciate that stopping when you are just satisfied is a way of honoring your body.

More Body Factors That Affect Weight

The body factor . . .

The cures to use . . .

5. Problems digesting too much carbohydrate.

You may have insulin resistance, which causes the body to be inefficient in clearing large amounts of carbohydrate from the blood. This may lead to further weight gain. This factor typically lessens or disappears with weight loss.

Balanced Eating and Mastery Living

Use Balanced Eating, but eat 3 rather than 2 servings of protein foods per day. Choose unrefined carbohydrates, such as 100 percent whole wheat bread rather than white bread. In addition, exercise daily 60 to 90 minutes.

6. Differences in fat cells.

You may have more fat cells than lean people. Gaining weight early in life or in pregnancy prompts fat cells to develop. Once you have a fat cell, it may not go away and may only shrink so small.

Body Pride

Use the Body Pride cure to honor and accept your body at a weight above that which you would otherwise prefer.

The body factor . . .

The cures to use . . .

7. Low sensitivity to signs of hunger and satisfaction.
You may have differences in the factors that regulate feelings of hunger and satisfaction. These differences may make you less accurate in knowing when your body needs you to start and stop eating.

Balanced Eating and Good Health
Use external signals such as weight loss to determine whether or not you are eating the right amount. Consider the risks and benefits of taking drugs to control your appetite.

the weight would resolve his diabetes. However, this latest news was not different from other jolts that had prompted Stanley to make major commitments to change in the past, only to be stalled by serious difficulties in following through.

Stanley needed to see for himself what had caused his weight problem, and now his diabetes. He also needed to examine the roots of his lifestyle patterns. In Stanley's case, before he could even think about the six cures, he needed to understand the origins of these patterns in his own life. I told him that with a simple test, he could predict the scores he'd have on the Solution Inventory well before he took it.

Stanley learned from the tests that his parents were rather responsive until the "year out of hell" in which the family home burned to the ground and three of his four grandparents died. With all the stresses, his parents became emotionally distant, but his father indulged them with toys and their mother appeased them with sweets.

Both he and Kristin continued the pattern of indulging themselves with food, but Stanley deprived himself in other areas. He pushed himself to become the admired doctor in the family and felt overwhelmed with stress. Kristin chose a different path. She was brighter than her brother, but underachieved. She indulged herself by staying with a mundane job that used only a fraction of her talents.

Is your pattern depriving, indulging or both?

Before you use the Solution Inventory to assess your skills in the six cures, let's take a few minutes to predict what those scores will be. Since these skills are learned, we had to learn them from someone. Typically we learn them from our parents, then continue to treat ourselves as they did. As a result of these influences, you developed a style of relating to yourself. If you have weight concerns, that pattern is typically permissive, depriving or a combination of the two.

What is a permissive style?

Permissiveness usually involves parenting that is overly close and indulgent. Contrary to what permissive parents might think, it is *not* nurturing. True nurturing means giving children what *they* need, not what parents need to give them. Permissive parents set few limits with their children, and when they do, their expectations are too low. They often don't check to see if the children followed through and see that the children suffer the natural consequences of their actions.

When we are indulged by others who respond with kindness when we are rude and heap us with accolades for a job poorly done, we learn that we can get away with things the real world would never allow. In the moment, being indulged is easier than toeing the line, but in the long run permissiveness leads to pain, failure and disenchantment. Not only will the world not baby us the way our parents did, but we don't develop a thick enough skin to face that reality. Later, when confronted with accurate feedback and lack of success, we feel confused, disappointed and hurt.

Permissiveness has many roots. Most parents who are permissive had permissive parents. Others had depriving parents and became permissive as an opposite reaction. Sometimes permissiveness occurs when parents, for whatever reason, feel guilty about a child. Permissiveness can also occur when parents have not separated from their own parents and learned autonomy. Such parents may be so enmeshed with their child—so overly close—that they feel the child's hurts, making it difficult to exert discipline or punishment. One look at the child's sad face and they withdraw their request to pick up the wet towels on the bathroom floor. What's more, when a parent relies on a child for emotional support, setting limits means potential rejection and loss of that closeness. Few of us would risk losing our chief source of companionship and love.

Keep in mind that although permissive parenting *looks like* excessive kindness, it always has a flip side that is abusive. One can only pick up the wet towels from the floor and listen to incessant whining for so long without the truth coming out. Yet because those honest feelings have been withheld, when they do emerge they are hostile, judging and shaming. Afterwards, guilt-ridden, the parent returns to indulgence.

A permissive relationship with ourselves . . .

Children of permissive parents often continue to treat themselves in a permissive way as adults, a pattern that does not serve them well.

> Donna, who raises Arabian horses in the rolling hills north of San Francisco, was the adored only child of older parents. "It sounds extreme, but all I had to do was frown a little and my mother would feel so sad and guilty that she'd give me my way. I still live with my parents on their ranch, and I'm happy, but I have a sense that I've never grown up. That's why food is so important to me. I've never been able to stay on diets, because eating a big dinner at night and having candy at bedtime makes me happy. I don't exercise, because I don't enjoy it. I'd rather sit on the couch and read a good book or watch a few videos."

Please use the self-test below to assess if you have a tendency to be *permissive*.

Is your style permissive?

yes no   1. I expect too little of myself.

yes no   2. I often feel the feelings of others more than I do my own.

yes no   3. Others claim I am oversensitive at times.

yes no   4. When things are difficult, I don't push myself.

yes no   5. I often feel powerless.

Is your relationship with yourself *permissive*?

yes   somewhat   no

What is a depriving style?

If permissiveness produces a relationship with *too much* closeness, giving and acceptance, then deprivation means having *too little*. Depriving parents don't give us enough nurturing. Without closeness and attentiveness early on, we're unlikely to know how we feel and what we need. We may even feel invisible. In depriving environments, limits are nonexistent, which leaves a child feeling unsafe, or so harsh that success is unlikely. The child is left feeling discouraged or rebellious.

One of the reasons depriving parenting is so destructive is that we are left feeling so *alone*. In fact, on an emotional level, we *are* alone. Because no one has planted within us a nurturing inner core and a sense of our own value, our inner voice is harsh and critical. As a result, our expectations of ourselves and others are unrealistically high and we are repeatedly disappointed. There is no soft cushion of love to fall back upon. External comforts—such as food—beckon.

Like permissiveness, deprivation has many roots. Parents may be absent physically or emotionally. Divorce, addictions, poverty, incarceration, work or traumatic events may separate parents and children. Even when parents are present, loving and willing, deprivation may still occur. Differences in personalities, a lack of early bonding or marital problems can all drive a wedge between what parents want to provide and what the child actually receives.

The deprivation we bring ourselves . . .

The legacy of childhood deprivation is long. We typically become our own harshest critic or let go of all disipline and plunge into a life of indulgence. Carl, a tire store manager, is someone who continued the pattern of deprivation into adulthood.

Carl's father spent most of the year on the road as a salesman, a job that neither paid well nor gave him pleasure. All his unhappiness was expressed when he was at home through being a strict disciplinarian with Carl. The marriage was a lonely one for Carl's mother, and she suffered bouts of depression that were severe enough to require occasional hospitalization. As a result, Carl was left alone a lot and was expected to help out in raising his younger brother.

By the time he came of age, a style of deprivation was well entrenched in his inner life. Carl's relationships with others were distant, but he was busy. He focused his attention on getting ahead, making money and amassing savings. According to Carl, "Life has been good to me. I have a good job and a good income. I really have no complaints. I'm pretty big and I've never married, but those things don't bother me."

Carl summarily wrote off many of life's deepest pleasures: intimacy, love and caring. It never occurred to him that he was perpetuating the pattern set by his father. The combination of growing up in emotional isolation and later adopting his father's harsh, critical inner voice made intimacy unlikely for Carl. His inner critic surfaced in every new relationship, scaring away any fledgling feelings of love or caring. It was almost inevitable that Carl would turn to food when emotional support was scarce.

Is your style depriving?

yes no   1. I expect too much of myself.

yes no   2. I often distance myself from my own feelings and those of others.

yes no   3. Others claim I am insensitive at times.

yes no   4. When things are difficult, I continue to push myself too hard.

yes no   5. I like to be in complete control.

Is your relationship with yourself *depriving*?

yes   somewhat   no

Again, please answer the questions on the previous page to assess your tendency to be *depriving*.

Our style is often mixed.

Parenting is often mixed—some permissiveness and some deprivation. Quite understandably, it's common to develop a mixed pattern within ourselves as well.

There are many variations on this. Parents may try to balance each other, with one taking the depriving role and the other the permissive one. Or one or both parents can have a variety of mosaic patterns of depriving and indulging themselves. Common examples are parents who are indulgent with the child but depriving with themselves or parents who seesaw between indulgence and deprivation, the strict disciplinarian becoming the soft marshmallow. Another pattern is clear deprivation in some areas—for example, work—and equally clear indulging in others—perhaps in eating, watching television or drinking.

> Susan complained of wide fluctuations in her weight, and as it turned out, she treated herself permissively in some ways and deprived herself in others. She was raised by an indulgent mother who periodically was harshly critical of her. Susan's dad was distant and depriving because of a drinking problem. She was so gifted in all arenas that she sailed through high school and college with honors and never had a shred of a problem until she decided it was time to settle down and marry.
>
> It was then that her combination of permissiveness and deprivation affected her weight and her life. Each potential partner brought up intense fears. Her permissive side worried she'd surrender to him and lose her power. On the other hand, her depriving side was so self-critical that she had no confidence in her ability to love a man well and so judgmental that nobody was ever good enough for her. As romances became closer, Susan's fears rose and she ate with abandon.

Is your style permissive, depriving or both?

Predicting the causes of your weight problem . . .

After reflecting on your style of relating to yourself, apply that information to predict your patterns with the six causes of weight problems. For each cure, find the pattern that best describes you.

Parenting Styles and the Six Cures

How we were parented as children and how we have parented ourselves as adults:

	Permissive	Depriving	Responsive
Nurturing	indulgent	depriving	responsive
Limits	too easy	too harsh	reasonable
Body Pride	false	critical	accepting
Good Health	excessive	inadequate	appropriate
Balanced Eating	indulgent	depriving	balanced
Mastery Living	chaotic	neglectful	balanced

Your Solution Inventory

Now that you have a greater understanding of the factors besides the six causes that impact your weight, take a moment to do what Stanley and so many others have done: develop your own personal profile by completing the Solution Inventory.

You will find that you score higher in some areas than others. In areas with high scores, you already have a strong base of skills. Mastering this method will only enhance them. However, the areas with lower scores are the more important causes of your weight problem. The cures that correspond to these causes will be especially important to concentrate on.

Many strengths and many opportunities . . .

To discover your personal strengths and opportunities, please total your score for each cause. The range for each cause is 0 to 9, and the range for the entire inventory is 0 to 54. The lower the score, the more that particular cause is likely to affect your weight. As you master the method, your scores will increase.

The Solution Inventory

Please circle the number that best describes how often you do each of the following:

	always	often	sometimes	never
1. Strong Nurturing				
I am aware of my feelings.	3	2	1	0
I recognize and meet my needs.	3	2	1	0
I ask for help from others.	3	2	1	0

Total ____

	always	often	sometimes	never
2. Effective Limits				
I set reasonable—not harsh or easy—expectations.	3	2	1	0
My thoughts are positive and powerful.	3	2	1	0
I face difficulties and follow through anyway.	3	2	1	0

Total ____

	always	often	sometimes	never
3. Body Pride				
I put myself down on account of my weight.	0	1	2	3
Being overweight helps me in certain ways.	0	1	2	3
I honor and accept my body.	3	2	1	0

Total ____

	always	often	sometimes	never

4. Good Health

I notice how healthy my body feels.	3	2	1	0
I take good care of my health.	3	2	1	0
My health care is effective.	3	2	1	0

Total ____

5. Balanced Eating

I eat regular meals.	3	2	1	0
I eat only when I am hungry and stop when I am satisfied, not full.	3	2	1	0
My food is healthy and pleasurable.	3	2	1	0

Total ____

6. Mastery Living

I am physically very active.	3	2	1	0
I engage in activities that are meaningful.	3	2	1	0
I take time to restore myself.	3	2	1	0

Total ____

The lower the score, the more this cure will help you solve your weight problem.

Building on Your Strengths

Now you can construct your own profile of the six cures. Begin by finding at least three areas that represent your highest scores and write them in the space below. These are your strengths.

My Strengths

1. _____

2. _____

3. _____

Next please find the three areas with the lowest scores, the areas you consider to be your biggest challenges and your biggest opportunities. Please write them below.

My Opportunities

1. _____

2. _____

3. _____

Revisit this inventory as often as you like as you experiment with the six cures. As it becomes easier for you to stay in balance, eat healthfully and live in an active and fulfilling way, you may be approaching your solution. At that point, be sure to use this self-test again to fully appreciate all that you have accomplished.

By the way, Stanley had predicted with his pattern of both depriving and indulging himself that he would find his biggest opportunities in Strong Nurturing and Effective Limits. That was just the case, and he had several strengths in the body and lifestyle cures.

Stanley now understood his weight problem and was primed to begin solving it, except for one thing. Even though he was a physician, he still needed to take a few minutes—as you will have opportunity to do in the next chapter—to decide if solving his weight problem was worth the trouble.

The question is, "How much does my weight matter?" Responding to that question is the next step toward your weight solution, and the answer is a very personal one.

How Much Does Your Weight Matter?

Tabloids can trumpet as many stories as they like about alien abductions, the headlines that really excite the public's imagination usually have to do with Oprah Winfrey's weight. This remarkable woman possesses beauty, wealth, talent, love and meaning in her life, but all that really matters to the public is the size of her body.

Weight doesn't hold much water.

Unfortunately for Oprah and the rest of us, a lean, firm body continues to be a touchstone in our society for weath, beauty, power and love. An angular jaw, a tight tummy and narrow hips

---

The decision to lose weight is personal. Consider . . .

How does weight affect my health?

What is the impact of weight on my happiness?

Do those effects *matter* to me?

---

signify that we possess certain admirable personal qualities, namely moral strength and physical vitality.

Of course, the cultural assumption that extra pounds signify lack of those qualities is patently false. People with weight problems expend, on the average, the same number of calories in physical activity as the lean and mean. Even when they are gaining weight, the average excess of calories consumed amounts to only 50 per day. *Fifty calories!* Surely eating the caloric equivalent of an extra *half apple* per day doesn't sound like a health sin or make us morally lacking.

The judgments about being overweight in our culture are simply expressions of *weightism*, fallacious beliefs that discredit people because of body size. Weightism is as pernicious as racism or sexism and it is even more universal. Moreover, studies have revealed that those with weight problems hold *even more* negative attitudes toward people of size than people of normal weight.

How can I be *objective* about my weight? The rest of the world isn't.

When there is *so much* riding on the number on the scale, it is nearly impossible to see our weight objectively. And we *do* need to see it objectively to deal with it effectively.

Becoming fully aware of what extra weight costs us in terms of health and happiness makes it possible for us to find our weight solutions. Only when we fully recognize the personal costs of our excess weight—neither exaggerating nor minimizing—can we decide whether or not our weight *matters* to us.

Mary, a 58-year-old real estate agent, was numb to her weight. She shrugged off her size even as her doctor, husband and friends nagged at her incessantly about how unhealthy she was becoming. How could Mary address her weight with singleness of purpose under all this pressure? Her weight seemed to be more important than she was, and everyone seemed to assume that her losing weight was their decision, not hers.

So Mary held on to her weight as if to her very survival. Yet by reacting to others instead of responding to her own views, she was unable to look her weight problem in the eye and answer the question "Is this really what I want for myself?"

"I love you *so much* I want to control your body size."

Often relatives and friends disrespect our decisions about weight in the name of *love*, and try to coax us, punish us or shame us into peeling off pounds. How insulting and ineffective! Body size is a very private and very personal decision.

Should friends, family and co-workers fail to respect your right to weigh whatever you choose, your task is clear. You need compassionately and persistently to guide them to *stop* trying to control your weight. No noticing what you eat, commenting on your body or lecturing you to exercise. No threatening or disapproving glances when you reach for seconds. The subject of weight must become untouchable.

Further, these loved ones must stop thinking they know more about what is right for you than you do. Your body size is *your* business alone. Only *you* know what is right for you! As the voices of others are quieted and the struggle for control ceases, you will then be able to hear your own true thoughts and feelings about your body size.

"I need you to keep your thoughts about my weight to yourself."

Carol was wildly successful in her household cleaning business—but her weight continued to increase. One evening she stepped out of a hot bathtub laced with peach oil and billowing with bubbles, feeling content and relaxed. She was still pink-skinned from the heat of the water when her husband, Ben, burst unexpectedly into the bathroom. He was startled to see her, but then said, "When are you going to lose weight? It's a shame. You're so beautiful. Why do you keep that weight on, anyway?"

Carol's anger flared. Fortunately, she had thoroughly digested the notion that her body was her own and the weightism of others was their problem, not hers. Carol took a deep breath and said, "Ben, I understand you want me to lose weight, but my weight is my own business. I need you to keep your thoughts about my weight to yourself. I need your acceptance that I will make my own choices about my weight."

It was only after this confrontation that Carol separated enough from Ben's preferences about her weight to make her own personal decision about her body size. A week later her weight began to drop.

"I know you mean well, but my weight is my own affair."

Bruce's weight markedly increased when he was promoted to assistant vice president of his firm and began to travel more frequently. His wife, Nancy, was in an emotional tailspin, worrying that his weight would affect his health. This anxiety climaxed during the couple's romantic getaway to Southern California.

They were enjoying a candlelit dinner at an elegant restaurant. Bruce had consumed three drinks, a prime rib dinner and half a basket of bread. Nancy stifled her criticism. However, when Bruce ordered a chocolate sundae with extra whipped cream for dessert, Nancy, red-faced and almost surprised by her own fury, launched into a lecture: "You're just digging yourself into an early grave with your eating. I don't think you care about us. It doesn't matter to you, does it, that you're letting down your family?"

Bruce quickly and effectively stopped Nancy's intrusion into his decisions about his weight: "Nancy, I know you mean well and I can see you're upset, but my weight is my own affair. I need you to back off about it." It was only then, when Bruce was able to feel psychologically alone with his weight problem, that he began to take it seriously. Was this how he wanted to live? Was overeating the way he wanted to receive his satisfaction? Was this the body he wanted for himself? Was it?

"I'm so mad at you for judging me, I'll stay heavy."

The most common reaction to feeling intruded upon and disdained because of our weight is to *stay heavy*. We express our outrage by holding on to our extra pounds as a way to retain control. In fact, keeping others from controlling us can take on more importance than attending to our own health and happiness. Ironically, our desire to prevent others from controlling our body size ends up giving them the ultimate control over how much we weigh.

Drawing a circle around yourself.

In my earliest years I relished playing dress-up and carrying my miniature purse stocked with red candy lipstick almost as much as I did making forts in the dusty vacant lot at the end of our street. This magical patch of ground offered hills for digging tunnels, and weeds for basking in. More important, it contained the loose dirt and finger-thick sticks the other neighborhood kids and I needed to define our turfs.

One scorching summer day, my brother and I were digging in the vacant lot and he kept throwing shovelfuls of dirt on my patch of ground and into my tunnel. I tolerated it for a while, but he persisted, until at last, thoroughly exasperated, I picked up a crooked stick, drew a deep line in the dirt and said in the most threatening voice a 5-year-old can muster, "That's it. I've *had* it. *Stop!*"

Does your weight matter?

If you pick up such a stick, trace a line around your entire body, and say to society, friends and family that when it comes to your weight . . .

> *"That's it. I've had it. Stop! I won't tolerate the pressure, the comments, the glances and the judgments anymore."*

. . . you will give your weight solution a stunning boost. By fending off the messages of others, you will be able to peer inward and ask with a fresh curiosity, "Does my weight matter *to me*?" Just because your weight is on the high side doesn't mean it's a problem. Weight is a problem only if it interferes with your health and happiness in ways that matter to *you.*

"My life does not revolve around my weight."

Danielle and her best friend, Linda, are the same height and weight. They take an early morning walk together, and if you were to ask them, they'd say they're very much alike. "We both have teenage daughters, we both have creative jobs we love, and our husbands are both football fans. We think and look so much alike we could be sisters." Yet the meaning of their weight is completely different. For Linda, those extra pounds mattered; for Danielle, they didn't.

Danielle has a life that despite mundane annoyances and obligations is for the most part fulfilling. She loves her husband deeply and still finds him romantically exciting. Her daughter, Ann, went through a rebellious period two years ago, but now Danielle enjoys a solid friendship with her. Danielle also has a wide circle of friends.

Her eating is reasonably healthy, except for periodic affairs with the cookie jar. She's in good shape for a person who spends eight hours a day at a computer terminal. No one in her family has had any weight-related health problems such as heart disease, high blood pressure or diabetes. Given her fulfillment in life, her family history and a healthy checkup, it is clear that Danielle's extra pounds are not a major issue.

"Weight is the major issue in my life."

Linda, on the other hand, has experienced some serious disappointments in her life. Though she loves her husband, their bedroom activities have been on the blink for more than three years. Moreover, the emotional tone of their relationship has been flat for some time. They don't enjoy spending time together, because they always fight. And Linda hasn't felt physically attractive or sexually desired for years.

What's more, Linda says, "I can't stand my obsession with food! I hate having to think about it all the time. I know every fast-food place that's on the way from home to my daughter Brigitte's school. I'm like an addict with french fries, cheeseburgers, bagels and lattes."

Linda's cholesterol level is high, and her father had high blood pressure and diabetes. It's clear that Linda's weight threatens her health and happiness.

Who says your weight is high?

The health risk posed by your weight is based, in part, on your height and weight. The heavier you are for your height, the higher the medical risk. The question becomes, to what extent, if any, are you overweight?

On the next page is a weight chart that will help you determine if your weight is high. Even if your weight *is* high, it doesn't necessarily mean it diminishes your health and happiness. Also, there are limitations to the value of the number on the scale. People of the same height and weight vary a great deal in how much of their weight is fat and how much is muscle.

Find your height in the left column, then locate the column in which your weight falls. That is your extent of overweight: low or none, medium or high. The ranges do not suggest that a weight gain within the "low or none" weight range is healthy. The higher weight within that category is only for people who have high levels of muscle and bone.

Body s*hape* changes the health risk.

The shape of your body also affects the health risk posed by your weight. You've probably heard that if you're shaped like a pear, weight isn't as much of a medical risk as if you're shaped like an apple, right? But do you know why? Whether you are an apple or a pear or somewhere in between, you need an explanation. Here it is.

When you carry your weight higher on your body (apple-shaped), it is more likely to surround the internal organs in the abdomen. Fat cells in this area of the body more readily release fatty fragments (free fatty acids) into the blood. More fat in the blood (triglycerides) means a higher risk of heart disease. More fat in the blood also makes it harder for muscles to burn blood sugar.

With extra sugar in the blood, the body secretes more insulin in an attempt to clear the sugar from the blood. These high levels of insulin in the blood trigger diabetes. Furthermore, the body reacts to having more insulin in the blood by absorbing more sodium, which increases the risk of high blood pressure.

For this reason, the higher you carry your weight, the more likely it is for the fat on your body to increase your risk of early

Your Amount of Overweight*

height	weight		
	little or none	moderate	high
4'10"	91–119	120–139	140+
4'11"	94–124	125–142	143+
5'0"	97–128	129–146	147+
5'1"	101–132	133–150	151+
5'2"	104–137	138–154	155+
5'3"	107–141	142–161	162+
5'4"	111–146	147–166	167+
5'5"	114–150	151–174	175+
5'6"	118–155	156–178	179+
5'7"	118–160	161–182	183+
5'8"	125–164	165–187	188+
5'9"	129–169	170–191	192+
5'10"	132–174	175–200	201+
5'11"	136–179	180–204	205+
6'0"	140–184	185–209	210+
6'1"	144–189	190–218	219+
6'2"	148–195	196–222	223+
6'3"	152–200	201–229	230+
6'4"	156–205	206–237	238+
6'5"	160–211	212–242	243+

* Derived from U.S. Department of Agriculture, Agricultural Research Service, Dietary Guidelines Advisory Committee. 1995. Report of the Dietary Guidelines Advisory Committee on the Dietary Guidelines for Americans, 1995, to the Secretary of Health and Human Services and the Secretary of Agriculture.

Where do you carry your weight?

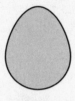  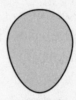

low
weight mainly
on hips, buttocks
and thighs

middle
weight in
both areas

high
weight mainly
on stomach
and chest

heart disease, high blood pressure and diabetes. It may also increase your risk for some kinds of cancer, although the ways it affects the development of cancer are not well understood.

To determine the shape that matches your body, just look at your silhouette in a full-length mirror and choose the shape from those above that is most similar to your own. *Low* means that you carry weight mainly on the lower parts of your body, *high*, in the upper parts of your body and *middle*, on both the lower and upper parts.

You can't choose your relatives . . .

Along with your size and shape, your health and the health of your relatives influence the risk of extra pounds. The diseases listed below can all be caused in part by obesity. Being overweight may make them worse. If you already have one or more of these conditions, a few extra pounds on the scale may pose a medical concern for you. And if any of your blood relatives have one or more of these conditions, extra weight is even more of a health risk because most diseases are in part influenced by genetic history. You may be more apt to acquire conditions that run in your

Conditions that make weight more of a health risk . . .

diabetes	gout
high blood pressure	difficulty breathing
stroke	loud snoring
heart attack	daytime sleepiness
angina (chest pain)	joint or bone problems
high cholesterol	arthritis
low HDL cholesterol	various cancers:
high triglycerides	uterus, cervix, ovary, breast, colon or prostate
gallbladder disease	

Do you have these conditions? Do your relatives?

family. A family history of heart disease, for example, would make your weight more of a medical concern.

Smoking plays a role.

The combination of smoking and being overweight, particularly when body fat is carried high or in the middle, is very risky. Smokers with upper-body obesity have a sevenfold increase in heart disease. Smoking seems to encourage fat to rest on the upper body, which increases the risk of heart disease, high blood pressure and diabetes, adding further to the health risk incurred by smoking.

Now put all this information together. On the next few pages assess the risk your weight poses to your health and happiness.

The comfort of having a little extra flesh

Fresh out of college and waiting for my husband to finish basic training at the tail end of the Vietnam War, I

The Risk to Your *Health* of Your Weight

	1 point	2 points	3 points
1. How much extra weight?	small	moderate	high
2. Where do you carry your weight?	low	–	high
3. Are you healthy*?	yes	–	no
4. Are your relatives healthy*?	yes	–	no
5. Do you smoke?	no	–	yes

* Healthy is having none of the health conditions
listed on page 126.

Scoring

To score each question, use the number at the
top of the column. Total your score and find
your risk category.

Your Total Score	Your Health Risk
5	low
6 – 9	moderate
10 or more	high

If you score "low," weight loss may improve your
health a little. If you score "moderate" or "high,"
losing weight may have greater health benefits.

Is weight a low, moderate or high risk to your health?

rented a room from Mrs. Sohaney, an elderly lady, and her wheel-chair-bound daughter, Helen, in Radcliffe, a little town in Kentucky, just outside Fort Knox.

Both women could have pulled in their belts a few notches. Mrs. Sohaney's blood pressure was a little high, and Helen was at times a little short of breath from being out of shape. Yet it was abundantly clear that these ladies were very happy. They belly-laughed at their favorite television programs, took daily walks and fussed over their periodic excursions to church, the doctor or the grocery store.

Their midday meal was the high point of their day, and almost always consisted of meat and potatoes, canned peaches or pears and little chocolate candies for dessert. All in all, they were content.

How much happiness is *enough*?

For Mrs. Sohaney and Helen, their weight was not keeping them from anything they wanted in life, nor did it expose them to any unusual health risks. If they had lost weight, they wouldn't have joined a line-dancing group or taken up tennis. Both liked their life just as it was. Was the happiness they'd gain from losing weight *worth* their giving up their familiar, pleasure-packed foods? Only they could say.

To guide you in considering to what extent, if any, losing weight will add to the happiness of your life, please respond to the questions that follow. When you are done, score your questions to estimate the limitations that extra weight might impose on your happiness.

Putting it all together . . .

Now you can see the extent to which weight blocks your health and happiness. The next step is to determine if those differences matter to you. Weight is a problem only if it affects your health and happiness in ways that *are important to you*. How happy and healthy you want to be is a personal decision. Please take a moment and reflect on what you've discovered about yourself in this chapter.

The Risk to Your *Happiness* of Your Weight

		little	some	much
1.	My weight depresses me.	1	2	3
2.	Thinking about weight makes me hostile.	1	2	3
3.	Staying overweight helps me not have feelings.	1	2	3
4.	My weight allows me to be passive, to hold back.	1	2	3
5.	Because of my weight, I feel less important.	1	2	3
6.	My weight makes me feel less attractive.	1	2	3
7.	I avoid certain sports or hobbies due to weight.	1	2	3
8.	I avoid some social situations because of weight.	1	2	3
9.	I would have more friends if I weren't heavy.	1	2	3
10.	My weight harms my close relationships.	1	2	3
11.	My weight detracts from my sexual fulfillment.	1	2	3
12.	My weight holds me back from earning more.	1	2	3
13.	I have work problems because of my weight.	1	2	3
14.	My weight keeps me from making life changes.	1	2	3

Points

Total Points

Scoring

To score each question, simply use the number at
the top of column. Total your score and find
your risk category.

Your Total Score	*Your Happiness Risk*
18 or less	low
18 – 25	moderate
26 or more	high

If you score "low," your happiness may not increase
as you lose weight. If you score "moderate" or
"high," weight loss may add to the joy and
fulfillment of your life.

Is weight a low, moderate or high risk to your happiness?

First think about your health. Is your level of health and vitality what you want for yourself? How would losing weight affect
your health and vitality? Does that greater amount of health and
vitality *matter* to you?

Next consider how happy you are now. Is that amount of happiness what you want for yourself? How much happier would you
feel if you cured both the symptom of weight and the underlying
drives and tensions? Does that extra amount of happiness *matter*
to you?

All in all, does your weight *matter* to you?

YES   NO

If your weight does not matter:
Please put this book down and do something else
that guides you toward even greater health and
happiness.

If your weight matters:
Please go on to the next chapter, continuing
your journey toward your personal weight
solution.

You Can Do This: It's an Inside Job

Every diet you have ever tried was an *outside* job. It asked you to *shape up* and *act right* externally: eat those carrots, drink that milk and by all means skip the butter, regardless of your inner yearnings and desires. *The Diet-Free Solution* is an *inside* job, a method of honoring and responding effectively to our inner selves, so that healthy living is a natural extension of vitality and balance in the mind, body and spirit. The yearnings and desires that detract from your health and happiness fade.

Yet if the solution is *internal*, how does one *go inside* so a solution can occur? In this chapter, I will share with you the experiences of others who have become comfortable with going inside themselves and allowing their solution to begin.

It's an inside job.

Your weight problem will be solved by achieving balance in mind, body and lifestyle. That is not done by a surgeon or a shrink. It is done by you. And the way you do it is to go inside yourself.

Cooling the desire for Belgian chocolates. It's an inside job.

Darcy was a tall, dark-haired woman who loved being the center of attention. She had a hearty laugh, a love for loud clothing and gold jewelry, and a formidable collection of western boots. She was the owner of a café that featured an unusual but successful combination of country and western singing and rich French food. When I met her she was desperate to lose weight and had tried everything: fasts, pills and 12-step programs, to no avail.

"Diets go against my nature because I'm a person who loves to eat. I'm someone who can wave good-bye to her friends as they go on a long hike, and stay behind picnicking on imported cheese, fresh French bread, white wine and my favorite Belgian chocolates. As long as I have this drive to eat too much, and this distaste for exercise, I know I won't ever lose weight and keep it off."

Darcy was absolutely right. How could she expect herself to change her *outside* actions—by, say, joining a gym and going on a diet—without changing her *inner* drives? In a sense, doing an outside job on weight is like trying to fix a stalled car by washing it and rotating the tires. The result is predictable: no matter how much effort goes into the washing and rotating, the engine will still refuse to turn over. Likewise, no matter how often Darcy forced herself to "act the part" by going on hikes or denying herself Belgian chocolates, her inner desires persisted and her weight problem would not be solved.

It's only when we *pop the hood* that a true solution can begin.

The solution to starting a stalled car begins by popping the hood. With access to the car's inner workings, tiny adjustments can be made to the engine that will allow the motor once again to run smoothly. Solving a weight problem, like fixing a stalled car, requires popping the hood and looking inside.

We become like the ace mechanic with a small bag of powerful tools—the cures—who regularly checks the engine, listening for noises and using those little tools to make small adjustments.

The car gets all the fine-tuning it needs and we enjoy a smooth ride toward our weight solution.

> ### *We become like an ace mechanic who enjoys a smooth ride.*

I watched Darcy as she began "popping her hood," looking inside, then making very small adjustments by asking herself the questions of the cures. She talked about the small adjustments she made—mainly in her thinking—as she used the six cures.

"I just pop my hood and go inside without any fear at all and see myself pulling out my tools and adjusting those harsh, negative thoughts and those impossible expectations and those absurd excuses about my eating. I calm right down and feel right in balance again, and those Belgian chocolates—I don't even care about them."

Darcy never did hike, but she did begin jazz dancing and karate lessons. After so many liquid diets, resolutions to exercise and bottles of diet pills, there was no question that what worked for Darcy was viewing weight loss as an inside job.

Going inside becomes a vacation you take many times a day.

If weight loss is an inside job, the question becomes: how do you *get inside* yourself? Tapping into your inner life is actually very simple, although the concept of it, and the practice of doing it, are rarely taught in Western societies.

Although going inside regularly throughout the day may seem odd or awkward at first, eventually it can become as easy as slipping into a well-worn bathrobe and fuzzy slippers. Going inside not only connects you with your thoughts and feelings, but also becomes another way of pleasuring yourself. The voice inside is supportive, safe and helpful. Looking inside is like a vacation you take, not once a year, but many times a day.

Once your awareness is inside, you ask yourself the questions of the cures. Each cure involves three questions, and after using one or more cures you will feel more balanced. You can then keep your fingers on the pulse of your inner life but otherwise go about your business of living.

What you will discover is that in this balanced state of mind, body and lifestyle you have achieved by going inside, your actions will be more purposeful, effective and satisfying.

A burning desire for chocolate cookies . . .

Let me walk you through a situation where I use the method of going inside to avoid emotional overeating. Sometimes while working at my computer, my mind drifts to a kitchen drawer containing a fresh package of really disgusting chocolate pinwheel cookies, the kind with the chocolate on the outside that looks like paint and tastes like plastic. They are one of the comfort foods from my childhood so, despite their flavor, I savor them. Every once in a while an intense desire to have these cookies arises in me. I know I'm not hungry, so I journey inside to find out what it is that I really need. In this case, asking myself the questions of the first cure, Strong Nurturing, is all I need to restore my inner balance and prevent overeating. These are the thoughts and feelings I experience as I journey within.

Step 1. Let go of your external life.

Right this minute I want a pinwheel cookie. I want at least one pinwheel—maybe two—so much, in fact, that I can already see myself going downstairs to the kitchen to find them. I consciously shut out the noise from the street and the sight of the pile of journals on my desk.

Step 2. Cross your boundary.

I know I need to go inside but I feel a little afraid. What will I find there? OK, go inside. That is where your power is. I'm a little uncomfortable, but that's OK. I take a deep breath and cross the boundary to my inner life.

Step 3. Ask yourself the questions of the mind cures.

I first notice a few thoughts: "I want the cookie. I deserve it. They aren't that many calories. I didn't eat a big lunch today." I let them pass and go a little deeper to where the feelings are. I'm

To Go Inside Yourself:

1. Let go of your external life.
Cut off from your thoughts and the cares of the day, consciously taking a mental vacation from them.

2. Cross your boundary.
In the blink of an eye, pass the boundary into your inner life. As you do, fears may arise, but they will fade.

3. Ask yourself the questions of the mind cures.
With curiosity and compassion, begin asking yourself the questions of the nurturing limits cycles until you feel balanced.

4. Ask yourself the questions of the body and lifestyles cures, if needed.
If you are not yet in balance, use the body or lifestyle cures until you are in balance once more.

5. Return to your external life and take action.
Continue to be aware of your feelings and thoughts. Return to your external life, and take any actions suggested by your inner journey.

not sure I can find any, but I wait and see, giving myself plenty of time.

I feel curious. What am I feeling, anyway? It should be interesting to find out. I wonder what hodgepodge of feelings I will find inside—both positive and negative. Although I enjoy the positive feelings more than the negative, I value both. The negative feelings will help me determine what I need. Just experiencing a negative feeling—giving it the full attention it deserves—can often relieve me of it.

How do I feel?. . . Guilty about my taxes. I haven't done them yet. I feel . . . restless because I've been sitting at the computer too long and I feel a little bored. I have been formatting charts all day and I'm tired of it. I need . . . to call my accountant and to take some exercise, perhaps a walk. Do I need support? No, not really. I can meet these needs by myself.

Step 4. Ask yourself questions from the body or lifestyle cures if needed.

I feel back in balance, so I don't need to check my body and lifestyle further.

Step 5. Return to your external life, and take any actions suggested by your inner journey.

I turned off the computer, changed into my running shoes and walked out the door for a brisk 3-mile walk. When I returned, I checked in with myself again, now feeling positive and relaxed. I called my accountant to arrange an appointment, then settled back to my work at the computer. Thoughts of the chocolate pinwheel cookies in the kitchen drawer downstairs had long since passed.

In the chapters that follow, you will see precisely how to make these cures work for you as you journey inside yourself. For right now, consider only the entry point into your weight solution, the process of going inside.

Common Reactions to Going Inside

In our groups, we make it clear that the skill of going inside is *absolutely central* to your weight solution. That usually stirs up a lot of reactions, questions and thoughts, which I will share with you now.

"I don't know if I have an inside."

Linda was a school counselor with a big family who had the largest blue eyes I have ever seen. Her life was very busy and full. As our group began strengthening their practice of going inside, Linda said to me, "Laurel, I don't know if I have an inside."

Of course Linda had an inside. This warm, giving woman had a husband and children who loved her, needed her and to whom she gave tremendous amounts of emotional and physical support. She was so busy noticing and responding to everybody else's needs that she rarely allowed herself the room to notice her own inner life.

"Linda, you are not empty. Fortunately, taking inner journeys will help you understand that. The more you go inside, the more aware you will become of the richness that was within you all along."

"Why don't I do this naturally?"

Another patient, Steve, found inner journeys frustrating. They just didn't come naturally to him, and he asked me, "If this is so important to do, then why doesn't it come naturally?"

Looking inward and checking what is inside oneself can be a very natural event. The only reason it didn't come naturally to Steve was that early in life his parents had taught him to do the opposite—that is, to focus on the outside.

Like most concerned parents, Steve's mother and father wanted him to succeed in life, and to them the external measures of success were what mattered. They rewarded Steve for flawless grades, perfect manners and the choir voice of an angel, and Steve took pride in trying to please them. Unfortunately, his parents' marriage began to fail. In his early teens, a dropped dish, a burned dinner or an unexpected bill would send either of his parents into emotional hysteria.

In Steve's view, all that was keeping his parents happy and together was their connection to him, and more specifically, the badges of success he wore: the grades, his concerts and his compliant behavior.

With his accomplishments so pivotal to the family's survival, it was no wonder that the idea of going inside himself and honoring his own feelings and needs was frightening. What if he wanted to play football rather than sing in the choir, and slack off on his grades a little so he could enjoy a normal teenage social life? Could he act on the feelings he found inside? It was no wonder that checking his inner life wasn't at all natural to Steve.

"How do I remember to go inside?"

It's not easy to remember to go inside. If you are used to focusing on getting the job done, making things happen and reaping satisfaction externally, then remembering to detach from the external life, move your awareness to within and notice the feelings and thoughts you find there is very difficult.

Yet people can learn to go inside in response to various prompts, including feelings, thoughts and situations. A chart describing common ones appears later in this chapter. Some people use normal daily activities to trigger their shift from the outer world to their inner life.

Steve remembered to go inside by using the normal routines of the day as prompts. He described it this way: "I check inside myself when I wake up, every time I eat, every time I go to the men's room and when I go to sleep at night. That amounts to about ten times per day, which seems to be enough to keep me in pretty good balance."

For others, external signals to take an inner journey—a wrist alarm, a bracelet, a rubber band around their wrist or notes by their telephone or refrigerator—give them a needed reminder to turn from the demands of the day to the world inside themselves. Typically these triggers are needed only when people begin using the method. Eventually the immediate benefits of going inside begin to motivate them to go there without a reminder.

"How do I know if I'm doing it right?"

It was important to Linda to be sure she was doing it correctly.

"How do I know if I'm going inside myself in the right way? Sometimes I'm not sure that it's my feelings I'm feeling or my husband's. Other times I don't think I get inside, but just hit the surface and stop there."

For Linda, it was a relief to learn that she *didn't have to do it right*. It was enough to use the method at her own pace and in her own way. There is plenty of leeway in using inner journeys; they are so powerful that people still reap tremendous rewards through using them imperfectly. Linda journeyed inside in her own way and still mastered the method well enough to solve her weight problem.

"But I'm afraid to go inside."

Of course you're afraid to go inside because you are venturing into what may feel like unknown territory or treacherous terrain. After years of going inside, I still find myself resistant at times, usually when I am out of emotional balance. I wish my whole miserable mood or embarrassing behavior would go away, so I wouldn't have to go inside myself and deal with it.

At those times, I try to remind myself that the fear of going inside is *just* fear, a feeling that passes. So I take a moment, watch the fear and sit with it. It doesn't feel good, but finally the fear fades. Then I give myself a mental shake, even though some residual fear remains, take a deep breath and go inside anyway.

"What if I can't find any feelings?"

That's fine; eventually you will. But if you are a thought-oriented person—one who reacts first by thinking, then later by feeling—you may find it more effective to start with the limits cycle. Many people find that if they process their thoughts first—which is what the limits cycle does—their awareness of their feelings immediately increases and they can then use the nurturing cycle with success.

Steve found that to be the case. "I never could reach my feelings directly. My thoughts were so strong that I couldn't get past them. So I tried using the limits cycle first and it had the effect of clearing away my thoughts. My feelings then were very apparent to me. Now I almost always use the limits cycle first and don't have a problem accessing my emotions."

"The voice inside me is not nice."

Paul was a wealthy man from a prominent San Francisco family. He had always had a bit of a paunch, but it had never bothered him in the slightest. However, when Paul was 37, his father, the adored and portly patriarch of his large Italian family, dropped dead of a heart attack. The day after his father's funeral, Paul started investigating ways to take care of his own weight and soon found our group at the university.

In our work together, two things surprised me about Paul. One was how quickly he mastered the cures. During our visits, he could easily go inside, ask himself the questions of the cures and achieve inner balance. The second was that he didn't lose an ounce in the first six weeks of his visits, for an interesting reason. Although Paul used the cures during our visits, in his own day-to-day life he didn't use them at all.

Paul: I don't use the cures because I don't want to go inside. It's not pleasant in there.

Laurel: You do it in our sessions. Is it unpleasant here, too?

Paul: There you help me with it and I hear it from your accepting perspective. When I'm on my own the voice is critical and negative, like my mother's voice.

Laurel: It sounds as if you need to find a loving, accepting voice inside yourself. You need a voice that is fair and honest, but kind.

Paul: I could use my father's voice. My father didn't spend a lot of time with me, but he liked me. When he looked at me, there was pride in his eyes. I could try using his voice instead of my mother's.

Paul began using his father's voice as a bridge until he found his own warm and positive inner voice. When he did, his weight plateau broke, and to his amazement, the scale showed a steady weight loss. The times when his weight did plateau again or when it increased were always when he returned to hearing his mother's harsh, critical voice inside. In time, he became more skilled at noticing when he was using her voice, and then he was able to return to his own warm and accepting inner tone.

If the voice inside you isn't warm and naturally accepting, it's not your fault; most of us carry inside of us the voice of one of the adults who raised us. However, it is essential that you create a relationship with yourself that is supportive and positive so that you will be more inclined to use the six cures.

If it's essential that you possess an inner voice that is positive, the question becomes, How do you get one? One way is very practical: *you borrow a positive voice until you develop your own.* Often the voice of a caring friend or compassionate relative is easy to slip into, but the voice of any famous figure you admire can also work well.

"You said feeling worse is progress?"

We can't live and grow if we feel numb. If numbness has been our most familiar state, then coming out of numbness is progress. However, when we emerge from the world of no feelings, both the positive and negative feelings come out. Although we haven't put out the welcome mat for the negative feelings, they arrive at our doorstep anyway. As a result, we may, for a time, feel worse.

Constance lamented, "I feel really scared and very sad. My feelings are so intense. What am I doing wrong?"

I told her, "Constance, feeling those feelings is *progress.* You are willing to stop being numb. And by feeling and releasing the bad feelings, you'll be better able to experience the good ones.

"Picture Noah's ark. Imagine good and bad feelings emerging like animals from the ark, in pairs padding down the ramp. As you feel and express the bad feelings, they will fade away. You can then round up the good feelings to enjoy for the remainder of your life."

This outpouring of emotion can be small or large, relatively easy or painfully difficult, and you may benefit from getting some help in expressing your feelings, including counseling. Yet inevitably this purging of the negative feelings will free you to be more spontaneous, more joyful and more alive.

"I was much more aware of my anger . . . "

Paul made an effort to find a more positive inner voice, and as he did he journeyed inside more often. What he became aware of was anger. Anger at his father for leaving him. Anger for his father's facade of a kindly philanthropist to the world, yet a rather stingy, withdrawn man at home.

In time Paul found those negative feelings enormously liberating. It had always bothered him that he had "no feelings" toward his father. Paul carried around a fair amount of guilt that he felt no affection for this man who was the reason for his financial good fortune.

However, once his negative feelings toward his father were released, Paul began remembering what was good about his dad: the chess games they played and the love of music they shared. For the first time he felt compassion and love for his father.

Meredith finally grieved.
It stopped her binge eating.

Another one of the people in Paul's group, Meredith, also felt worse when she journeyed inside. Her mother had died when she was 7. When Meredith entered the training, she was 42 years old and her daughter, Nicole, was 7, the same ages Meredith and her mother had been at the time of her mother's death. It was a frightening time in Meredith's life.

It became clear that Meredith had numbed herself with food for most of her adult life and had a genuine fear of going inside herself. For the first few weeks, she didn't go inside at all. She could sense that it was more than she could handle at the time. But seeing others in our little community go inside, surviving negative feelings and then reclaiming positive ones, encouraged her to make the journey too.

As Meredith began checking her feelings and thoughts she found she was sitting on a huge pile of rage. RAGE! She was furious at her mother for leaving her, and she was furious at her father for neglecting her. When her feelings were the most intense, I encouraged her to find additional nurturing and support from a therapist.

What interested Meredith most was that after releasing her negative feelings, her eating binges came to a halt. They stopped. During the following year, Meredith's angers and fears came and went, along with her willingness to experience those intensely negative feelings that constituted her first large step toward her weight solution.

"Did you say this becomes easier?"

Yes. Just like learning to pump iron or ride a bike, the more you do it, the easier it becomes. *So what* if at first you feel nothing inside? It doesn't matter that going inside feels a little awkward initially. So did going to work, falling in love and having sex. The first sense of awkwardness, embarrassment or resentment will pass away, and in time you won't feel as if you're faking it. Taking inner journeys throughout the day will be working well for you, and that is all that matters.

"How often should I take an inner journey?"

You should take an inner journey as often as you need to in order to stay in emotional balance. Some days you'll do it only a few times, and other days, far more often. There are no rules. The key is not how often you use this tool but that you go inside as often as you need to in order to maintain your inner balance most of the time. Linda and Steve used the method well but in very different ways.

> Linda enjoyed her newfound state of being aware of herself as a kind of continuous meditation. She drew strength from not losing herself to others and being vigilant about her own feelings and needs.
>
> Steve used a more structured approach, diving into the external world during his workday, yet regularly coming up for air to check out his inner life. He needed to get away from himself to focus on his work, but found that taking the inner journey every hour or two at specific times—before and after eating and exercise, on his way to work and his way home—worked best.

Your solution has already begun.

Already you understand the method, and even if only unconsciously, you have probably begun applying it to yourself. You may be finding that you are checking in with yourself more often throughout the day. *That alone may be enough to bring about your weight solution and lead you to the six rewards.*

When to Go Inside?

When you *feel* bad:
angry   sad   afraid   guilty   lonely   hungry
tired   sick   numb   depressed   hostile

When your *thinking* isn't effective:
thinking about food when you aren't hungry
thinking about weight when that isn't the problem
thinking about any one thing too much

When your *actions* involve too much:
eating, drinking, spending, working, sleeping, drugs,
overactivity, compulsive sex, reckless actions

When your *actions* involve too little:
pleasure, spending, working, sleeping,
social contact, exercise, sexual activity, interests

When the *situation* is difficult:
meals you tend to overeat
any vacation or work trip
social situations
situations that are emotionally charged

Anytime, to keep yourself in balance:
On rising in the morning. Going to bed at night.
In the shower or bathroom. Before and after eating

If you want to give your inner meanderings more power, ask yourself the questions of the cures. These are the tools to make you even more effective once you "pop the hood" to check your life within. If you want to make going inside yourself easier, lessen your inner stresses by writing the Thinking Journals and the Feelings Letters. The chapters that follow will help you do this.

That is all there is to solving your weight problem. You do not need volumes more information. Once you become accustomed to journeying inside often, you will naturally draw upon the strength, wisdom and goodness within . . . and that is more than enough.

Part 3
The Six Powerful Cures

For each cause there is a cure. When all the causes are cured, your weight problem will be solved.

Cure 1. Strong Nurturing

When I mentioned to Lynn, a petite and energetic nurse from Kansas who had only recently settled in San Francisco, that the first cure was Strong Nurturing, she was quick to interrupt me—not rudely, but with excitement because she thought she understood.

"I know. I should be good to myself. I'd love to do just that, maybe go on a shopping spree at Union Square or for a weekend in Carmel. But I can't. My husband, Jake, was just laid off his job in Silicon Valley. . . ."

Cure 1. Strong Nurturing

Effectiveness in getting your needs met.

3. Support   **1. Feelings**

2. Needs

Lynn looked glum. She had already decided that she could never lose weight because there wasn't enough money for shopping sprees or romantic getaways.

"Lynn, you have everything you need right now, even with Jake out of work, to nurture yourself very effectively—and not just once in a while but *every day, all day long.* You don't have to wait until you are on easy street and have a charmed life. You can live in a way that nurtures you right now."

Nurturing isn't a trip to Tahiti. It's an intimate, internal process.

Lynn wasn't convinced. "Jake has no job and I'm working swing shifts at the hospital. My daughter Karen just had her third ear infection this year, and all of my family and friends are back in Kansas. How can I be happy? How can I possibly keep from comforting myself with food?"

"Maybe you can't right now. That may be true. But you'll never know for sure until you embrace the tool of nurturing yourself. Nurturing is not what you think it is. You can't buy it, because it isn't something that's outside you. Rather, nurturing is a very personal internal process some people learn from the example of their parents as they are raised."

"My parents weren't nurturers. They were worried I'd be spoiled. . . . "

"It has nothing to do with being spoiled. It's a way of taking responsibility for yourself by tapping into the deepest part of you and determining what you need from the feelings that arise."

"I don't know what I need. I know what my parents need and what Jake needs. I don't even know if I want to know what I need."

"What happens is intriguing. When you start going inside, you find a virtual hotbed of feelings, some positive, some difficult, but all valuable because each of those feelings is deep enough to lead us in the direction of recognizing our true needs.

"Most people are amazed to find that their feelings vary from moment to moment, so much so that they understand instantly why they shut down emotionally and numb-out so often. By the end of the day there is such a pileup of feelings that no one could *possibly* sort them out and find their corresponding needs.

"But there is more. . . . "

Lynn continued to be intent, wanting the answer.

"The simple nurturing process—which amounts to asking yourself three questions—'How do I feel?' 'What do I need?' and 'Do I need support?'—is comforting in itself. Even if you don't discover your needs by doing it, just asking yourself those questions reduces your stress."

"Like when I have too many patients assigned to me and they're all angry and all I can think about is going to the candy machine during my break. . . . "

"Exactly, Lynn. In that case how do you feel?"

"At the hospital when I've been assigned six patients instead of three? Angry, rushed, frustrated . . . "

"What do you need?"

"Candy."

Unfortunately, like most of us, Lynn had learned to use food as her entire emotional vocabulary. When she was tired she ate, when she was lonely she ate, and when she felt angry she ate.

"You want candy, but what do you *need*? Candy fulfills your need when your body is hungry. What fulfills your need when you're angry, rushed and frustrated?"

"I don't know."

"Don't rush yourself. Just keep asking the question. Just keep going inside and ask yourself the questions 'How do I feel?' 'What do I need?' 'Do I need support?' Think of the way a devoted parent checks and rechecks a new baby every few minutes, wordlessly saying, 'How do you feel? What do you need? What can I do to help?' It's exactly the same."

Lynn was put off by my last statement. "Yes, but I'm not a baby. I'm 33 years old and have a child of my own."

"Think of it this way. If we don't treat ourselves as well as we would treat a child, we are at risk of feeling needy and are likely to start acting like children!"

"I am definitely not an adult when I go for the candy machine or flake out on the couch. I'd say I was acting like a 4-year-old with very long legs."

"That's exactly right! So even if you were the most mature adult imaginable, the truth is that you'd still need to be attended to, not by a doting mother or a devoted father, but by yourself."

"Actually, I think that's true," said Lynn. "If I treated myself with the same consideration and sensitivity I give to my 4-year-old daughter Karen . . . I don't think I'd be eating a pint of ice cream at 10 o'clock at night and I'd probably have the energy to take her for a bike ride after dinner rather than crash in front of the television all evening."

I nodded.

Lynn ran with this idea. "So nurturing myself does not necessarily mean indulging myself. If I bought flowers for myself, which I can't afford right now, I'd feel guilty and that wouldn't be nurturing to me. And if I slept until noon I'd miss my daughter Karen's softball game, and she'd be hurt, which would sadden me, not nurture me."

Ask yourself the questions of the nurturing cycle throughout the day.

"Precisely, and the only way you'll know whether or not what you choose to do will meet your needs is to ask yourself the questions of the nurturing cycle throughout the day. That way you'll be aware of your feelings because you're keeping your fingers on the pulse of your inner life. That degree of awareness will be key to figuring out what you need."

Lynn frowned. "I could probably figure out how I'm feeling, but I couldn't possibly know what I need. I mean, there's an endless list of needs I have. I've been collecting them for 33 years."

I had faced that same worry myself, so I understood Lynn's feeling of confusion. "You'll know. There is a lot of strength, wisdom and goodness inside you that will tell you quite accurately how you feel and what you need. That inner awareness is no different from your biceps."

Now Lynn was annoyed. "Biceps?"

"It sounds strange, but your skill in nurturing yourself is a lot like using a muscle. The more you work it, the stronger it gets. The more often you ask yourself how you feel, the more accurate your answers will be. The more frequently you think about what you need, the easier it will be to determine what your true needs are. Asking for support gets easier with practice too."

Using the cycles is like pumping iron. You get stronger and stronger.

"I don't ask for support. I take care of things on my own."

"I know. It's the most challenging part of the cycle, but it's also the most valuable. Nobody can meet *all* of their own needs *all* of the time. Life goes better for us when we ask for support. And making a request of another person creates intimacy. In asking for support, there is a soul-level touch between two people that is all wrapped up in vulnerability, closeness and autonomy. As you become even more skilled at making requests of others, I think you'll be amazed at their power to leave you feeling fulfilled."

"I don't often make requests of other people, because I think they'll judge me. How do I know they won't think I'm demanding or incompetent because I can't take care of everything myself? And I hate to be turned down. It leaves me feeling so foolish . . . and so unworthy."

Lynn was reacting the way we all do. There are risks in making requests, but what she didn't yet know was that there are safety nets built into the method. . . .

"My mother-in-law straightens every drawer . . . "

"You will feel more secure when you ask for support, Lynn, because the method has two safety nets.

"One is that if you become accustomed to using the words of the nurturing cycle (I feel . . . I need . . . and Would you please . . .), you automatically speak in an assertive way. The simple act of using those words will protect you from slipping into being passive or aggressive—that is, holding back so much that it hurts you or going too far and imposing on others.

"Second, soon you'll begin using the second cure, Effective Limits, to soothe and protect yourself when people respond to your requests in a negative way."

Lynn frowned. "It would never be safe to ask my mother-in-law for anything. She straightens every drawer in my house when she visits."

I laughed. "Good. You can send her to my house. There's nothing I'd like better!"

"She meddles in my affairs and tells me that I'm raising Karen all wrong."

"You're right, Lynn. She may not be safe to ask for support, but the limits cycle will help you determine that. But that comes later. Right now, you're mastering the nurturing cycle."

First you start with feelings . . .

Lynn was understandably anxious. "The only way I'll ever learn to do this is by doing it. I think I need to jump in and try it."

"Great. If you like, we can start now. How do you feel?"

"About what?"

"About anything you feel strongly about—either positively or negatively."

"My mother-in-law. She's coming to visit us for the holidays and I know she'll start cleaning my house as if I'm a sloppy housekeeper and telling me how to raise Karen."

"Good. Please try it again with the 'I feel' words, so you are better prepared to know what you need."

"I feel afraid that my mother-in-law will start giving advice and taking over as if she were the woman of the house."

"Excellent. That's just right. Any other feelings? Angry, sad or guilty? Anything else?"

"Yes. I feel angry about it too. How dare she treat me with such disrespect!"

Then you find your true needs.

"Great. You feel afraid and angry. What do you need?"

"I need . . . How do I know what I need?"

"Lynn, there's no need to rush. Just take your time and it will come to you. You may come up with several needs before you hit on the ones that feel right. Relax and just think about what you need."

"I need for her not to visit. Just the thought of her arriving makes me want to eat. It's not that she isn't a nice woman. She's Karen's grandmother and I do enjoy her at times, but it drives me crazy when she starts giving me advice about Karen, and then she starts rummaging through my drawers and putting everything in neat stacks. Actually, I could use some help cleaning, so that's not so much of a problem.

"What's really got me upset is that I know she's going to start lecturing me about giving Karen more discipline or cutting Karen's hair or giving Karen the kind of vitamins she buys. . . . "

Lynn paused and for a moment looked confused, but she took plenty of time before she continued. "Well, I guess what I really want is for her to respect me as a mother, to give her opinion but treat it like an opinion—not to treat me as though she is obviously the good mother and I'm a big disappointment."

Last, if necessary, you ask for support.

"You're doing great."

"There's no way I can meet that need. Forget it."

I listened to Lynn intently, remembering back to when I also routinely discarded a need before even exploring it.

"Lynn, just stay with the cycle. Work it through."

Lynn frowned, as if she were listening to herself for the first time. Then she cracked a smile. "I don't even take my needs seriously, do I? I don't have the conviction that I matter and that I have to pursue meeting my needs."

"You're getting more of a commitment to honoring yourself, Lynn. Just using the cycle right now will make you stronger. What you need now is to figure out what you need from your mother-in-law."

"Her name is Mabel. I need to ask her, 'Mabel, would you please talk with me about something that is difficult to talk about?'"

"Fabulous. Now use all three parts of the cycle so that she can receive the message you are sending. Use the words of the nurturing cycle: I feel . . . I need . . . and Would you please . . . ."

"I could say, 'I enjoy your visits and I'm happy that you're Karen's grandmother, but often when you're here, I feel angry when you tell me how to raise my daughter. You state your opinion as if you're right and I'm wrong. Would you please keep giving your opinions, but state them as opinions, not facts?'"

"Excellent. If you were to stop there, would you be in emotional balance?"

"I think so. I feel so much better not letting her treat me as if I were inferior. I feel much more in balance. There is no doubt about it."

"If you still don't feel in balance, don't drop the ball. Continue using the cycles until you have regained it. It's tempting to go around the cycle once and feel so relieved that you stop using it too soon. You end up abandoning yourself before you've regained inner balance."

Lynn picked up on this thought. "That's why the cures are cycles; you go round and round them intentionally until you are in emotional balance."

"Exactly."

"If I were passive, afterward I'd probably eat."

Lynn fell back in the chair and hooted, "I always gain five pounds when she visits. If I could tell her the truth like that, I don't think I'd be eating a whole pint of ice cream at night."

On her first use of the nurturing cycle, Lynn had calmed herself down, returned to emotional balance and been able to assert and meet her needs about a very sensitive and complex matter.

Later, she reported back to the group that she had successfully saved herself from eating the nightly pint of ice cream for the five nights of her mother-in-law's visit. She said, "It didn't require willpower. I didn't jump all over her aggressively. I just noticed my feelings and needs, and when I needed her support, I asked her for it. This stuff really works."

Developing this powerhouse of a skill is what you will do through this chapter. I'll show you all three parts of the cure. You'll see that what Lynn did wasn't hard at all and that you probably do it often already without even thinking about it.

The Nurturing Cure, Part 1— *How do I feel?*

One day when my son Joe was 12 and experiencing a surge of adolescent separation, we were chatting in the car and he mentioned a disagreement he'd had that day with his best friend. Being one who often teeters on the edge of intrusiveness, I responded far too eagerly, "How do you feel about it? How do you *feel*?" He looked at me, his face screwed up in that wince teenagers reserve exclusively for their mothers, and said, "Feelings! Feelings! *Stay out of my feelings!*"

At that tenuous point in his flight to manhood, Joe couldn't share his feelings with me, only his thoughts. It didn't matter if Joe's thoughts were as jumbled as a messy closet or neat as hangers lined up evenly on the clothes rod. Sharing his thoughts kept me at a safe distance, whereas sharing his feelings would reveal far too much of his inner core.

The nurturing cycle's role is to honor our emotional essence. Since feelings run so much deeper than thoughts in our internal landscape, the cycle begins by checking our feelings.

Why do feelings have to be so difficult?

Since feelings are so important, it's a shame they're so difficult to locate, decipher and manage. In the first of our group sessions, I ask patients to describe their usual feelings. The most common reactions are:

"I have only one feeling. Hunger."

"I'm a rational person. I'm not good at feelings. In fact, I'm not sure I have any."

"I have nothing but feelings. I'm angry, sad, frustrated, guilty, afraid, disappointed, discouraged, jealous, lonely. . . . "

"There are big ups. There are big downs. And there is nothingness. There is nothing in between."

Recognizing feelings is difficult for many reasons. Perhaps our early training didn't validate our feelings, or we've developed an unconscious defense against feeling them, or we fear they'll explode like a volcano and we won't ever recover.

It's no wonder that as adults most of us can balance the checkbook, unload the dishwasher and wash the car, yet few of us have mastered the infinitely more important skill of recognizing our feelings.

The nurturing cycle will build this skill into your repertoire. Right now you may bait your hook and fish for feelings within, only to come up empty-handed. Or perhaps you come up with a thought instead of a feeling. Feelings can be hard to catch. They tend not to travel in straight lines but rather to swim at different paces and in different directions.

The two fears about feelings . . .

There are two frightening things about feelings: tapping into them and not tapping into them. If we tap into them, can we manage the feelings? If we ignore them, will they emerge in other ways that harm us?

It's far better that we tap into them. If we possess the courage to bring up feelings and tame them with the nurturing and limits cycles, we'll have some control over them because at least we'll know what is there.

How do I feel . . . ?

Approach all feelings with curiosity and compassion.
All feelings are valuable, even the ones that are difficult.

You will have many opposite feelings.
It is normal to have many feelings, often opposite ones, at the same time.

Don't worry about getting it right.
The feelings you don't recognize now will arise again later on.

Separate feelings from thoughts.
Notice the thoughts that masquerade as feelings such as "I feel *that* . . . " Continue until you find the feeling underneath the thought.

Filter out smokescreens.
"Stress" and "upset" are not feelings. Continue exploring until you find the true feeling behind the smokescreen.

Find a balance of good and bad feelings.
Look for balance, if it is there: the hint of anger behind the calm or the joy that bubbles up through the depression.

Check that the feeling and need correspond.
Rearrange the emotional crossed wires within you. For example, sadness suggests the need to cry, not to eat.

Become skilled at feeling a feeling and letting it fade.
Allow a feeling to come over you—*to really feel it*—and then watch it fade.

If we don't, the feelings we ignore come back to bite us. In my early days at the university, Marna Cohen, a kindly, wise social worker, took me under her wing. One afternoon during an intense conference about how to manage a depressed adolescent patient, she explained to me how the feelings that we push down never really leave us.

"If feelings aren't expressed, they go underground only to come up later, with a much bigger wallop. Not only will the feelings be stronger, but they'll show themselves indirectly, making them harder to uncover. When the feelings are cloaked in eating, spending or drinking problems, it's easy to focus on the outward difficulty rather than getting at the root causes, the unexpressed emotions."

There are myriad examples of this dynamic. The hurt from being teased for not measuring up in sports may resurface as an affinity for television. The sadness that results when a loved one dies can go underground and later rear its head as a powerful urge for chocolate. Anger about body rejection by a parent later appears as an unconscious drive to maintain a large body size.

Quietly and repeatedly asking yourself "How do I feel?" is a way to slowly—at your own pace and in your own way—uncover the buried feelings that may be causing your appetite to soar or your body size to stay at a level above your genetic comfort zone.

Bait the hook. If you don't pull up feelings, rebait it.

It's perfectly fine to check your feelings and come up empty-handed. You've still done something very important because the act of going inside with curiosity and compassion is nurturing in and of itself. If at first you don't find the feelings inside, continue to ask yourself how you feel until the feelings surface. Or, if you prefer, wait and then rebait the hook to check your feelings out later.

Katherine, a public defender, often felt caught between two images of herself: the good caring lawyer and the bad food junkie. She had difficulty finding both her positive and her negative feelings because she not only didn't trust feelings, but judged them. When she was angry, that was a bad feeling. She pushed it aside. When she felt happy, she felt insecure. Why would she be happy? If she was happy now, when would the feeling stop?

Raised by strict German parents, she developed excellent work habits, but little compassion for normal human feelings, including her own. It was much easier for her to stay in the familiar world of thoughts. Yet Katherine's nightly eating binges gave her a clue that she had to begin to understand her own emotional world. She knew it wasn't the pasta and ice cream she wanted, but she had no idea what she did want. Her answers, as Katherine well knew, were reflected in her feelings.

According to Katherine, "I'm getting better at approaching my feelings with some curiosity, as if to say, 'What feelings are in there now?' I can't wait to find out, so I can use that information. If it's hate, so what? If it's anger, good. Likewise if the feeling is gratitude or joy. I'm not making any judgments about them. All my feelings are important."

Watch for thoughts that masquerade as feelings.

There is absolutely no way you can do the nurturing cycle wrong. However, several ideas can help guide you.

One pattern that diminishes the nurturing cycle's strength is mistaking thoughts for feelings. Nearly any sentence that beings with "I feel *that* . . . " is probably a thought.

Another is to use smokescreens. Smokescreens are words that sound like feelings but are so nonspecific that it's virtually impossible to tell what the real feeling is. If we don't know what our basic feeling is, how can we determine our need with any precision? For instance, if I realize I am tired, it's not hard to figure out that what I need is rest. Yet if I label that tiredness as *stress*, I don't know if I need to scream, to sleep, to cry or to exercise.

Often when we say we are stressed it's because there is a veritable pileup of feelings and it's difficult to tease them apart. We must, however, for by separating our various feelings, we gain the power to identify and meet our true needs. So although there is nothing wrong with going inside and coming up with a smokescreen or nonspecific feelings, finding a basic feeling will help you more directly determine your actual need.

The thought	An actual feeling
I feel . . . she was wrong.	I feel angry.
I feel . . . there is no hope.	I feel sad.
I feel . . . that I'm lazy.	I feel guilty.

Lynn did well. She expressed her feelings and avoided smokescreens.

As a nurse practitioner in a city clinic, Lynn's patient load was tremendous. She had lobbied her boss for more time at the end of the day to chart patient records and return phone calls. Instead of responding to her request, Lynn's boss had added four hours per week to her clinical caseload. Lynn's first reaction was to feel hungry and think about going to the cafeteria. Instead, she used the nurturing cycle: "*I feel . . . stressed out. I feel . . . bad. I feel confused. What I really feel is angry. Really angry!*"

Instead of grabbing for external solutions—the candy or the chips—Lynn's simple maneuver, to pause and check her feelings, resulted in her realizing that in fact she wasn't hungry at all. In fact, she had just eaten lunch!

Yet if Lynn hadn't stopped and taken an inner journey to find the basic feeling, she would have headed to the cafeteria. Not only would she have eaten food her body didn't need, she would have distracted herself from her true feelings—and been unable to find and meet her actual need.

The smokescreen	Could be many feelings . . .
I feel stressed.	I feel tired, guilty or afraid.
I feel upset.	I feel angry, sad or guilty.
I feel bad.	I feel lonely, sick or hungry.

As it turned out, Lynn determined that she needed to meet with her boss to discuss the situation. She made an appointment to see him the next day. In addition, she needed to seriously consider looking for a position with a more reasonable workload.

You will often dig down to some very basic feelings.

Just like Lynn, you too will get better at identifying your true feelings.

David, an insurance broker, after losing six pounds in his first month using the method, found that his weight stabilized for two weeks. After talking to his fiancée, Stephanie, he realized he was simply eating too much food. He'd thought he could eat freely because the foods he was eating were healthy and he worked out for an hour a day at the gym.

The next day before leaving his office to buy his mid-morning bagel, David paused and asked himself: "How do I feel?" Bad. I feel like . . . eating. I'm sick of eating when I'm not really hungry. Why do I want the food? How do I really feel? I feel fed up with working and not getting paid enough. I feel afraid I'm never going to get out of debt. I feel guilty for having gotten myself in this situation to begin with.

When David dug down to his basic feelings, he found a whole spectrum—from anger to fear to guilt. What a relief. At least he knew what he was really dealing with instead of interpreting his feelings as hunger. Each feeling pointed to a need that, at the very least, could be examined and considered, if not met.

The bagels stopped being the enemy and weight stopped being the problem. What David began to focus on was restoring his inner balance, in part by recognizing his feelings and needs. This was the start of David disconnecting from the external solution of food and trusting enough to go inside himself and tap into the wisdom, goodness and strength that was there.

Both Lynn and David were able to identify their basic feelings, the ones that provide us with accurate information to use in determining our needs. These basic feelings can be positive or negative, and experiencing a range of them is the essence of emotional balance.

The satisfaction of earned rewards

Experiencing these basic feelings keeps us balanced, true to ourselves and growing. They are the nourishment needed for a dynamic, meaningful life. Positive feelings are our earned rewards, encouraging us to continue to meet our needs.

When you call a friend and she's happy to hear from you, there is an immediate payoff, an earned reward. That burst of warmth and pleasure reinforces you to pick up the phone to call that friend again. In time, you develop a circle of friends who bring a little sunshine into the day. As a result, life is better.

The Basic Feelings of Emotional Balance:

Earned Rewards	*Essential Pain*
grateful	angry
happy	sad
secure	afraid
proud	guilty
rested	tired
satisfied	hungry
loved	lonely
well	sick

The lessons learned from essential pain

Negative feelings, the essential pain, are the blaring sirens and flashing lights that tell us that our behavior has not served us well. If we can feel this pain, rather than escape it, we can rapidly learn to choose a more fruitful path next time.

Consider the typical parent who comes home from work to a house full of screaming kids. The parental *suicide hour* of the day.

The habitual response? To escape the pain of the noise and commotion by diving into a feast of a dinner. However, the price we pay for not fully feeling that essential pain is to continue the same pattern. Instead of unlocking the motivation to make the situation better, we keep coming home night after night to screaming kids and overeating.

As you routinely dig down to the basic balanced feelings, you may notice patterns. Just the way some people like sweets while others like savories, your emotional pattern may lean one way or the other—toward the very positive or the very negative emotions.

The positive feelings were difficult to find.

For instance, Lynn tended to get stuck in negative feelings. She seemed to always be sad, angry, lonely or afraid. When Jake bought her flowers after receiving a new job offer, she brushed it off. She was used to feeling bad and could not allow the good in her life to sink in. Feeling bad wasn't pleasant to her, but it was familiar. Lynn's challenge was to recognize this pattern and search out positive feelings. Only then could she establish true inner balance.

Negative feelings escaped him.

David's denial had two consequences in his life. First, blocking out his essential pain kept him from dealing with his weight, his overexercising and his financial problems. Second, because he lacked the balance that comes from feeling both earned rewards and essential pain, people sensed that he was not authentic. Many group members felt alienated from him, and few took him seriously as a potential friend. Being with him was unsettling, and people probably felt betrayed as we all do when we seek closeness with someone who never allows us in because they themselves are reluctant to look inside.

What proved helpful to David? To see his essential pain not as bad or wrong, but as quite valuable. David took very small steps, first shifting his attitude toward his dark feelings. He then began to check for his essential pain when he journeyed inside.

Our "crossed wires" can be uncrossed.

Another common pattern you might see in yourself as you use the cycle is "crossed wires." If you were raised by parents who weren't aware of their own feelings, they probably weren't accurate in recognizing yours. As a consequence, you may not have received all the direct and indirect messages you needed in order to know the difference between, for instance, feeling hungry and tired, or feeling lonely and sad.

The result? Crossed wires. You have one feeling, but interpret it as another. That sets you up for two missteps: filling a need you *don't* have, and leaving unfilled a need you *do* have. Common crossed wires are:

"When I feel tired, I think I'm depressed. When I think I'm depressed, I eat."

"I interpret anger as hunger. But it's a special kind of appetite, one that goes for something crunchy that I can bite into and tear apart."

"When I feel sad, I feel tired, and think I need to boost my energy with food."

"When I feel tired, I think I look ugly and fat, which makes me feel hungry."

The solution to crossed wires is to find the basic feeling. Usually what happens is that a need surfaces, often "*I need food.*" Pause and ask yourself, *"How do I feel?"* It's likely that you'll sense you aren't hungry at all. What you feel is, for instance, tired.

The remarkable power of simply feeling the feeling . . .

In addition to interpreting one feeling as another, it is common to have been taught that feelings either don't exist or are too overwhelming to tolerate. The net result in either case is the same. We never learned that *we can survive having feelings*.

However, with the tools of the method, you will soon learn how remarkably resilient you are. You will also learn that it is OK to allow difficult feelings to come up. They *won't* overcome you and you *won't* fall apart. The feelings will wash over you and begin to fade. If you are sad, stop everything and feel the sadness. Stay focused on the feeling of sadness without allowing powerless, negative thinking to drag you down into self-pity. If you are angry, feel the anger without letting thoughts plummet your emotions into hostility or rage.

What will happen? Chances are, like a bell-shaped curve, the sadness or anger will rise and fall. You will naturally return to emotional balance.

> Lynn loved to cook. She'd been raised on a farm, where the women made big meals at breakfast and dinner for the whole family. As a result, a big part of her identity was wrapped around family meals and the art of cooking. With Jake out of work, Lynn extended her nursing hours and the cooking chores fell on Jake's shoulders.
>
> She shared with the group a story about a difficult evening she'd had the previous week. Coming home from work, emotionally exhausted from having experienced the death of one of her patients, she had walked into the house and nobody had noticed her. Jake was preoccupied with his computer, and Karen was watching television. Lynn walked into the kitchen. Every plate was dirtied. She opened the refrigerator, the bread drawer, the cupboards. There wasn't an ounce of food in the house other than mustard, mayonnaise, ketchup and dried soup mixes. Lynn collapsed onto the sofa and cried.
>
> Jake heard her crying and approached her with concern. Karen, on the other hand, was impervious, glued to the television.
>
> Long slow tears ran down Lynn's cheeks. "Jake. I'm sad. I'm really sad. I miss cooking and I miss our little family dinners. Right now, this is all we can do. But it is still sad." Lynn cried a little more, but avoided dipping into self-pity and becoming depressed or blaming Jake and becoming hostile. She did not distract herself from

---

Feeling a Feeling Is:

- not stuffing it, ignoring it, or distracting yourself from it.

- allowing it to rise up in your belly, burn in your throat and saturate your being.

- waiting for it to naturally subside, which it will.

- knowing that afterward you will say it wasn't so difficult and that you are stronger than you knew.

---

the feeling by going to the cookie drawer. What Lynn did to maintain her inner balance was to use the very effective tool of feeling her feelings until they faded.

To add more feelings to the repertoire of those you are now able to feel and face, choose a new one. The next time it comes up, intentionally savor it like a wise observer who is compassionate and curious. You might say to yourself, "Oh, I feel afraid. I wonder if I can hold on to that feeling? If I do, will it fade naturally?" or "Gee, I feel hungry. I wonder if I can tolerate that feeling for a few moments and see if it subsides."

Then watch yourself feel the feeling; just as you experience the heat of a sunburn or the bitter cold of winter air. What if the feeling does not fade? What if it becomes more intense? There are many choices of action. One is to help it fade by using journals, Feelings Letters, counseling or prayer.

If that seems too difficult, you may not be ready to feel that feeling, which is fine, or your feeling may be too intense and require meeting your need. For instance, if you are still hungry ten minutes later, eat something. The point of tolerating all these difficult feelings is to enhance our resilience, given the reality that every day of our lives we will experience some of them. This practice of feeling the feelings and allowing them to fade keeps us from rushing too quickly to avoid them—such as distracting ourselves by overeating. Avoiding them also creates an inner cli-

Which Feelings Can You *Feel* and Let Fade?

angry	sad	afraid	guilty
tired	hungry	lonely	sick

mate of fragility. We live in a state of constant anxiety, anticipating our next discomfort and worrying that we won't be able to handle it.

As you are enhancing your skill at feeling these feelings and letting them fade, you may find that it is too difficult for you. If so, distracting yourself with healthy pursuits, such as exercise, the outdoors, a good book or even television, may be your best alternative. These distractions aren't bad or wrong, because you are on the right path and you are respecting yourself by going at your own pace. Keep practicing feeling your feelings—just as you would practice the piano or practice your golf swing—and it will become easier and easier in time.

The Nurturing Cure, Part 2— *What do I need?*

Now that you are skilled at recognizing your feelings, *what do you do with them?* You move to the second part of the cycle and decide what you need, just as David did after he mastered the skill of recognizing feelings. At first when David checked his feelings, he told me, "There's nothing there. No feeling. I don't know what I feel!"

I encouraged him, "You will, David. Just keep asking yourself the question and before long you will be surprised at how skilled you become at answering it."

By our next session David could answer the question with the words *bad, good, tired* and *nothing.* By the next week, he had added *angry* and *sad,* and by the fourth session, he could feel and express the entire range of feelings. Then he hit a roadblock.

"My mind goes blank when I try to determine what I need. I know what I 'should' need, what my parents told me I needed and what is socially acceptable to need, but what do I personally need? I'm not sure. . . . "

Meeting your needs when you are already in emotional balance

"When I'm angry, I usually need to get it out physically with a long walk or express it by writing in my journal."

"I was tired so often that I had to sit down and take some time to come up with a plan for how I was going to get to sleep at night."

"I was hungry. I needed to eat something healthy that would satisfy me without making me overly full."

"My basic feelings are being tired and anxious. What do I need? Something relaxing to do alone. I dig in the garden or work in my shop."

"I felt so stressed about work. My feeling was a balanced one, fear. I was afraid I couldn't do the work. What did I need? Not to escape or downplay the feeling, just to feel it. When I totally concentrated on my fear, it seemed to go away. I discovered I could do the work. The fear was my problem, not my ability to do the job."

Regaining your balance, then determining your needs

So you know how you feel and it isn't good. It isn't one of the basic feelings either. You're feeling not sad but depressed, not angry but hostile or not tired but completely exhausted.

What do you need? *To return yourself to emotional balance.* I can ask myself what I need when I'm depressed, and because I'm out of balance, my answer won't be very accurate. I'm too out of balance for that. As a result, when you are out of balance, it is important! Your priority must shift from the project or mission at hand to the pursuit of inner balance. Without that inner balance, nothing you touch will turn golden and little that you do will be fulfilling.

But how do you regain your inner balance? By using the cycles, particularly the nurturing and limits cures.

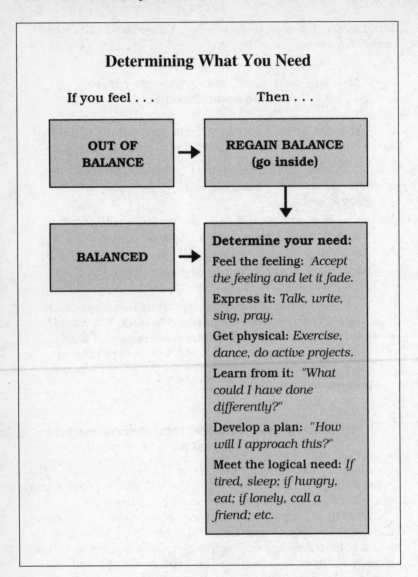

Determining What You Need

If you feel . . .   **Then . . .**

| OUT OF BALANCE | → | REGAIN BALANCE (go inside) |

↓

| BALANCED | → | **Determine your need:**

Feel the feeling: *Accept the feeling and let it fade.*

Express it: *Talk, write, sing, pray.*

Get physical: *Exercise, dance, do active projects.*

Learn from it: *"What could I have done differently?"*

Develop a plan: *"How will I approach this?"*

Meet the logical need: *If tired, sleep; if hungry, eat; if lonely, call a friend; etc.* |

Numb after work . . .

"After work I feel numb, and all I can think about is food. There is a certain joy in that, so I'd say I feel joyful and rebellious too. I know I'm not in balance. I go in my room and lie on the bed. I go inside using the cycles until

I find inner balance again. Sometimes it takes just a minute. Other times I need far more time. Once I'm in balance, I have my energy and my optimism back and I know right away what I need."

Powerless with Mother . . .

"I feel so powerless around my mother. She can cut me to the bone with one glance. Then I feel like a little kid again, wanting to please her but hating myself for giving in to her. I usually have to physically remove myself from the situation for a few minutes. I go to the bathroom and take a few deep breaths. I use the nurturing and limits cycles a few times until I'm back in balance. What do I need? Being around my mother is toxic to me. I need to be away from her for now."

A rebellious high . . .

"When I'm really on a high, I celebrate with food. I go into this fantasy state that is by nature rebellious and self-destructive. It's a false high and I know it's not going to lead anywhere but to a crash. I bring myself back into balance by checking my feelings and needs and using the limits cycle.

"What is my balanced feeling at that moment? A mixture of joy and anxiety. What do I need? To feel the pure feelings of joy and anxiety without doing anything, without distracting myself by eating. I also need to sit in the feelings until they fade. Why should I overeat when I'm joyful? All that does is give me indigestion and make me gain weight."

Being a "baby" about sickness . . .

"I rarely get sick, but when I do I go right into an unnecessary low. I don't only feel sick, but also powerless, depressed and furious. I get back into emotional balance with effort by using all the cycles, and when I do I find I need to allow myself to be as miserable as I want to be, for as long as I want to be. Somehow, allowing myself to be a complete baby about being sick is just what I need."

If this is Saturday, I must need time alone.

Each of these people has used the nurturing cycle to begin forming concepts about what they need. These general needs give us a shorthand, when we are out of balance, for finding our true need quickly. By completing his needs list, David learned several things about himself.

It was such a relief to say he was sorry . . .

David saw that he tolerated too much from people, then lashed out at them and, in the end, felt a wave of guilt about his snarly tone. He'd grown accustomed to carrying a cloud of guilt with him and he wasn't aware that he had chipped away at his sense of his own goodness. When he realized that feeling guilty meant he needed to apologize, he began to feel remorse and express it more often.

What he also saw was a pattern of feeling unbalanced after being passive and overly accommodating of others. It was really self-pity that he felt because others were taking advantage of him. David knew he couldn't pull himself out of self-pity until he first used the cycles to return to balance. Often what he needed once he returned himself to balance was nothing more than to develop a plan for how to do things differently next time.

There were other needs that David began to meet more effectively. Often he'd skip meals and ignore his hunger during the day. He learned instead to pay attention to his body and eat when he was hungry. He then found he was less hungry at dinner. In fifteen years in his business, David had missed only three days of work due to sickness. It wasn't that he didn't get sick but that he would work right through any illness. The idea that it was important to meet his need to stay home and in bed with chicken soup was new to David.

A defiant self-destructiveness cried out for balance.

The last entry on David's list was rebelliousness. For long periods, his behavior would be passive. He'd be too nice to his business partner, Diane, give up too much for his relatives and be overly generous with his friends. Then there would arise in him an intense rebelliousness that was defiant and self-destructive. But because he was such a warm and mild-mannered man, he expressed the defiance through binges—drinking beer and eating hot dogs to the point of feeling sick—and through reckless driving that had cost him two traffic tickets.

His need? To get back into emotional balance through the cycles, then assert his needs more in his day-to-day life. David was able to do this periodically. He did occasionally lapse back into passivity, but when he used the nurturing and limits cycles his driving became saner and his eating more balanced.

Lifting herself out of fear . . .

Meeting her own needs was a little more challenging for Lynn. She resisted meeting them in part because she felt a certain irritation that no one else could do this for her. It was so difficult to determine just what she needed, let alone push to get her needs met. Why couldn't Jake do it for her? *Why couldn't Jake make her happy?*

Facing that aloneness, that truth that only she could meet her needs, took time. Yet Lynn's resistance to taking on this responsibility was prompted by more than her desire to be rescued. She had been so deprived as a child that an inkling of an unmet need—for instance, Jake's loss of income—resulted in a full-blown panic that only food seemed to soothe.

As Lynn developed a list of her needs, she realized that when she was afraid, she could feel her fear and eventually it would fade. She didn't have to rush to eat something to distract herself. After the feeling faded, she could take action by coming up with a plan for doing what she could about their financial situation and letting go of the rest.

Lynn's need was to learn to tolerate a little hunger.

Moreover, Lynn noticed how sensitive she was to even a small twinge of hunger. Going hungry as a child had led her to interpret her hunger as threatening. What she needed was to feel her hunger without overreacting to it. Perhaps all she needed was a piece of fruit to quiet her hunger, nothing more.

Jake often said that what bothered him most was

when Lynn panicked about not having enough food or money. The panic would come over her unexpectedly, and Jake would immediately react with anger. *Why was she so afraid? Didn't she trust him?*

In the past, Lynn had reacted to Jake's anger by feeling more powerless and more frightened. As she used the nurturing and limits cycles to create a thicker emotional boundary, she no longer felt Jake's anger so intensely and could soothe her own fear somewhat. Once she regained a semblance of inner balance, Lynn could then ask herself, "What do I need?"

If she was afraid about not having the food she needed, she would pick up the telephone and express her fears to a friend, who quieted them. If her friend was busy, she would write in her journal, and that helped as well. When her panic was about money, expressing her feelings to her friend or through a journal didn't help Lynn. What helped her was sitting down with a calculator and making a financial plan. She also said a prayer, trying to have faith that things would work out as they should.

Lynn's need was to be aware of the good things, not just the bad.

Last, as Lynn used the journals and letters and emptied out some of her emotional distress, she became more aware of the good both in herself and in life in general. She had always brushed aside the good feelings in life—except for the pleasure she derived from food. Now she began to feel more positive feelings—pride, joy and contentment.

She needed to savor her pride about how she had mothered Karen, and the fine care she gave people who were sick. What's more, she was feeling more grateful for Jake and the family life they were building. It wasn't perfect, but it was so much better than what she had experienced as a child. Rather than holding her gratitude in, she needed to express it to Jake and tell him how important he was to her.

Becoming aware of your own needs . . .

You can begin the process of constructing your own list of needs. Just think of the common feelings that arise for you and what helps you meet the needs the feelings suggest.

Your Needs List

When I feel . . .   **I usually need . . .**

_____   _____

_____   _____

_____   _____

_____   _____

_____   _____

_____   _____

The Nurturing Cure, Part 3—
Do I need support?

The third and last part of the nurturing cycle is to ask yourself "Do I need support?" and if you do, to request it from others. It is at once the most difficult and the most rewarding part of this cycle.

When I began to be aware of how isolated I was in my "I'll take care of myself" attitude and to make requests of others, I felt inadequate, vulnerable and guilty for burdening them. Unconsciously I asked:

- What's wrong with me that I can't do it myself?

- What if the person I ask says no? Could I recover?

- What if they say yes when they really should say no, or give me support and then later resent me or punish me for it?

- What business do I have asking others to take my burden?

Making requests of others was just too treacherous then. It was easier to do everything myself. In time, it became a little safer for me. If someone said no, I could soothe myself and not take it personally. I was aware of my feelings, so if making a request of a particular person felt unsafe, I could pull back from making it.

My boundaries were a little thicker from using limits cycles, so I wasn't oversensitive to everybody's displeasure, feeling their pain before even they did! In any case, I couldn't do everything myself, and if I cared that my needs were met, I had to bite the bullet and ask!

Stepping off the pedestal . . .

Yet I still hung back from making requests, until I realized that what stopped me was a kind of arrogance. By not making requests I kept myself up on the pedestal of self-reliance, out of emotional reach from others.

As long as I *gave* and never *took*, I was in control. In the grand scheme of things, I didn't need people, so people couldn't hurt me. I maintained this false power by not telling people what I needed, by staying aloof. In reality, I remained a scared little girl terribly afraid of being vulnerable or being rejected.

Did I really want to see myself as arrogant, controlling, frightened and removed? No, not really. Thus began a growing devotion to making appropriate requests of others—as a reminder that I had indeed stepped off the pedestal, and as a statement to myself that I wasn't that scared, insecure, seemingly arrogant little girl any longer. I could need. I could receive. I could be grateful.

Serving up a hamburger sandwich . . .

I became aware of how often I felt like the 4-year-old with very long legs that Lynn had described, and I recognized that I wasn't alone. If I felt that way, maybe other people did too, including those from whom I requested support.

So even though I was more willing to ask and more ready to receive, I was painfully aware that I had to learn how to make requests so that others could hear me—yet still listen to themselves and not try to do more than they could do. That need required me to master the art of . . . *the hamburger sandwich.*

How much I needed that tool. I had buried my needs for so long that when they finally surfaced, my requests sounded demanding, ungrateful and even somewhat cold, without my realizing it. It was as if I delivered the request knowing full well that it probably wouldn't be met, that I probably didn't deserve to have it met and that even if it were met, it wouldn't be *enough*. In fact, I was already a little angry, even before my request had been answered!

Being passive and denying my own needs for so long had the perverse effect of making my requests unintentionally lop-sided—long on taking care of *myself* and short on taking care of the *other person*. I unknowingly neglected to show respect, consideration and gratitude to the person from whom I was requesting support.

There are many variations on this theme—such as expecting people to guess what we need and being hurt and withdrawn if they don't. Or expecting to be given the moon with little thought of giving back in return.

As you might surmise, people don't always take kindly to these patterns. The exchange leaves the relationship more barren, with less trust and less harmony. In my own case, I knew that my clumsiness in making requests held me back in many ways, but what was I to *do about it*?

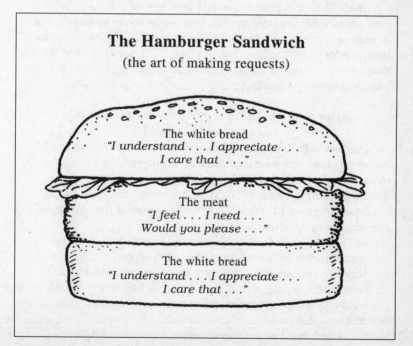

The Hamburger Sandwich
(the art of making requests)

The white bread
*"I understand . . . I appreciate . . .
I care that . . ."*

The meat
*"I feel . . . I need . . .
Would you please . . ."*

The white bread
*"I understand . . . I appreciate . . .
I care that . . ."*

I knew I needed to stay in assertion rather than wandering into passivity or aggression. I had to be able to state my needs while respecting theirs, using the words of the nurturing cycle: *I feel . . . , I need . . .* and *Would you please. . . .* But somehow it was clear that that wasn't enough.

Am I speaking to an adult or to a 4-year-old with long legs?

Perhaps if I were talking adult to adult, just using the nurturing cycle would be enough to engage the person, to make my needs clear and ask for support. But who can guess how the person we are making the request of is functioning right then?

Perhaps they are in their adult mode and can respond in a rational and balanced way. Or perhaps not. Perhaps they are out of balance and need to be treated the way we all need to be treated at times—like a child. This doesn't mean coddling them in a patronizing way, but giving them a full measure of understanding, respect and acceptance while we make our request.

Their chronological age would give me no guidance whatsoever about whether they were in their adult mode or feeling like a 4-year-old with long legs. So, to be safe and effective, it seemed only prudent to wrap the *meat* of *I feel . . . , I need . . .* and *Would you please . . .* in the *white bread* of expressing honest compassion and sincere empathy.

After living with his work problem for so long, David quickly solved it.

David had decided to talk with his business partner about their work arrangement. The current situation was a financial disaster for him, and with his impending marriage to Stephanie, it could mean economic troubles for his bride as well. What's more, the strain of the problem was always with him.

David was a tremendously kindly man and saw making requests as demanding, which had gotten him into this impossible work situation to start with. David practiced role-playing giving his partner a hamburger sandwich—that is, an effective request. He began with *I feel. . . .*

"I feel that our arrangement isn't working out."

"That's a good start, but let's switch that thought to a feeling."

David paused, trying to figure out his feeling. "I feel scared about my money situation. I need to change our working arrangement so I stop losing money. Would you please take back your accounts? I can't do more than my share anymore."

"Good, you gave her the meat of your message. How do you feel?"

"Bad. In fact, I don't know if I could bring myself to tell her that. The woman is very sick. I'd feel like a jerk."

"Let's try it again, this time adding white bread on each side—that is, truthful statements that are compassionate and caring and begin with the word I."

David cleared his throat, "OK. Diane, I understand how hard it has been for you and I wish you weren't sick. I care that you are OK financially, but I'm feeling scared myself. My income and my clients have dropped off since I started picking up your clients. I need to find a way to change our situation so I earn more money and so I don't feel like I'm deserting you. Would you please talk with me about it so we can come up with a plan that will work for both of us?"

"Fantastic. Now finish with more white bread, if you can."

"I understand this will mean changes for you, and I know what you're going through isn't easy."

"How do you feel now?"

"I feel pretty good. I could say that to her and I think we'd probably work some compromise out."

When David came to the session the following week, he was elated. He even stood taller. "I talked to Diane and I was assertive and gave her the meat of my message and plenty of honest compassion, plenty of white bread. She heard what I said and wasn't offended. In fact, she said she'd been feeling guilty about what I'd been doing. After living with this problem for nearly a year, we solved the problem rather rapidly. She'll pay me more of the commission and do some support work for me when she's not sick.

"So, it worked! And I lost three pounds this week. It's amazing how the weight drops off when my stress level drops."

Use the nurturing cycle to be assertive . . .

Assertive
"I feel . . . I need . . . Would you please . . ."

. . . and avoid the less effective patterns of being passive, aggressive, or alternating between the two.

Passive		Aggressive
Say nothing. Later act aggressive toward yourself or others.	←→	*"You are . . . You did . . . You must . . ."*

Lynn used the plenty of white bread with Jake.

Eating in the late evening is typically a sign of lack of intimacy. This was Lynn's pattern, including late-night chocolates, after-dinner bowls of ice cream and bedtime munches on breads. Lynn knew full well that her needs for closeness and comfort in the evening weren't being met.

"I feel . . . upset. . . . "

"Good. Keep going and find the basic feeling behind the smokescreen."

"I feel lonely at night. Lonely and tired and unimportant. Karen is asleep, Jake's in the study and I'm . . . alone and all I can think about is eating. I need to feel important and I probably need a way to unwind. I know I need to figure out ways to relax myself at night, but I also need Jake's attention then."

What Lynn said worried me because meeting needs begins with doing what we can for ourselves before we make requests of others. "Let's start with what you can do for yourself. What do you need from yourself to feel loved, rested and important?"

Lynn thought for a moment. "Quite honestly, I need some time. I need time to develop some interests that feed me without food. I work all day and there is more than enough housework and child care at night to keep me busy. But there is no time for me to become involved in activities that make me laugh or interest me intellectually. I love calligraphy and I never take time to do it. I have friends I never bother to call. I can start doing those things again.

"But I also want some closeness from Jake. Right now we have no evenings without Karen wanting attention, and no time for lovemaking. With a life as devoid of pleasure and relaxation as mine, who wouldn't overeat in the evenings?"

Lynn knew what she needed, but making a compassionate yet assertive request was completely foreign to her. Instead, she was familiar with holding back, then sinking into an unnecessary low—which then gave her more than enough emotional fire to be aggressive toward herself with the chocolate and ice cream or toward Jake by speaking to him in harsh tones. Her challenge was to stay in assertion—that is, to appreciate her own needs as well as Jake's.

Being passive, in the end, is no "nicer" than being aggressive.

The old adage "It's nice to be nice" is probably true, but being *too nice* is another story. The sum total of passivity—of rescuing others, giving too much and allowing too much to be taken from us—is no nicer than the angry stare, the dirty trick or the straight-out yelling of aggression.

Sooner or later we end up persecuting the person we've been rescuing. The lie about our true feelings can be maintained for only so long. When the truth eventually comes out, we turn our latent aggression toward others or toward ourselves—by overeating or a myriad of other acts.

It would have been *nice* for Lynn to accept that Jake would be less emotionally attentive to her because of all the turmoil from losing his job and having to seek new opportunities elsewhere.

On the other hand, it would have been *too nice* if Lynn had passively allowed Jake to neglect their relationship for so long that it cut into the basic fabric of their emotional bond. Lynn's overwillingness to ignore her needs was like setting a mousetrap that would spring sooner or later. The more Lynn pulled back the spring by rescuing others rather than making reasonable requests, the more certain it was that she would eventually erupt into aggression.

Lynn was well aware of her pattern. I inquired, "Lynn, why don't you ask Jake for what you need? For a minute, pretend I'm Jake and give me some nice warm white bread of understanding and caring to the extent that you can say it with sincerity. Then use the nurturing cycle to tell me your feelings and needs, the meat of the message, and last show consideration for me again with another piece of white bread. I know this sounds a little rigid, but try using the exact words of the nurturing cycle. When you express yourself through that framework, you reap far more rewards."

Staying on the intimate path of assertion

Lynn was willing to try it. "OK, let's see. Jake, I feel that you don't give me attention at night."

"You just did what we all do. Jake's important to you and this is a sensitive issue. So what happens? We revert to old ways."

"I get it. I told him a thought, not a feeling. I'll try I feel . . . again."

"That's where your power to connect resides."

Having the presence and skill to reach way down deep inside, identify your feeling and flat out say it has tremendous power.

Otherwise, if we don't state our feelings, we are inevitably stating our thoughts. Since each of us has any number of thoughts, the chance of finding a shared thought between two people is relatively slim.

On the other hand, all people have the same few basic feelings. If I say to you, "I feel sad that my marriage ended in divorce," you may never have experienced divorce but there is no doubt that you have experienced sadness. As a result, there is immediate empathy—the emotional connection that makes us more sympathetic to the requester's need. We are more likely to say yes.

Surprisingly, intimacy can be catching.

More important, opening up is contagious. By throwing out an "I feel . . ." it's as if we're casting a line into the water. We're welcoming the other person to take the tender morsel of our feeling and share an intimate conversation with us. In other words, in addition to receiving the support we desire, we receive the intimacy we need.

> Lynn cleared her throat. "OK, I'll go for it. 'Jake, I often feel lonely at night. I miss you. I need to talk with you about how we can spend some time together in the evenings. Would you please talk with me about it?'"
>
> "Very good. What would Jake say to that?"
>
> "He'd say, 'Not right now. Let's talk about it later,' and then not get around to it for a week."
>
> "Then you'd feel . . . "
>
> ". . . more unimportant, more lonely and more like eating leftovers from dinner. He can be so insensitive. I can't stand it."
>
> "How he acts is his choice. Your job is to stay assertive. Even if you don't get what you want, you've acted like an adult and been effective. That's using your power. Would you try giving him a hamburger sandwich?"
>
> Lynn nodded. "Jake, I love you and I want to be close to you. I understand that this has been a hard time for both of us. I feel sad because we don't have much time together, and I need some time to discuss with you what to do about it. If you can't take time tonight, I need your commitment to take some time tomorrow. Would you please give me

that? You are important to me and I understand you are rushed and pressured, but I need this from you."

"Excellent. You've stayed in assertion. You connected with him using the I feel . . . , I need . . . and Would you please . . . , and you gave him enough of the consideration and caring he needs to want to listen to you and meet your needs. You did a great job!"

In fact, Lynn had the same discussion with Jake after the meeting that evening. At our next group session, she reported on the results. "Well, I used white bread and I delivered my meat, and he agreed to talk. We talked that evening and I realized I needed cuddling from him and some listening. I don't think he recognized how essential that is to my day, and now he does. We haven't been perfect about taking that time, but we're doing it more and it feels so much better. I felt safer too because by using the nurturing cycle I knew I wasn't going to get aggressive or back off and do it my usual passive way. It gave me some structure, which helped."

Concepts from the nurturing cycle:
Lifestyle surgery

As you regularly bring up your feelings and meet your needs, you can't help but notice patterns.

"Everybody in my family likes hikes, but I don't. I go for a swim or catch up on paying bills while they do that."

"Sex is far more important to me than I realized, and I enjoy lovemaking more when I feel very clean and very attractive. So I take time for extra grooming."

"The holidays are so exhausting. What I really need is to go away on a little trip then, so now that's what I do."

"I know I'm supposed to enjoy vacations, but I don't. I prefer day vacations, little outings to museums or antiques shops, so that's what I do instead."

"On Saturday mornings I'm usually tired. I don't plan anything on Saturday mornings anymore."

In essence, you'll naturally create some patterns of external nurturing that work for you, which you may think of as *lifestyle surgery*. You clip away at the activities that don't meet your needs and substitute those that do.

This may sound like common sense, but often we do things because we *should*, it's *expected* or everybody *else* does. The nurturing cycle has created a direct pipeline to your inner life, so you now know how you feel and what you need. Whereas before you may have planned a vacation at the beach because *everybody* likes the beach, or gone to the Italian restaurant because *everybody* in the family likes Italian food, now you have narrowed the field to what *you* like.

Now, you'll find time to spend a day at antiques shops in the city or make it to a professional basketball game once a month simply because you want to. There doesn't have to be any reason for doing these things; just your desire to do them is enough.

For a while, you may need to fake it.

We all know that we'll never give up food for comfort until our lifestyle is nurturing. But what if we don't feel *motivated* to do lifestyle surgery that will bring us that nurturing, rewarding way of living?

You don't have to want to do it. Making your life better doesn't have to come from the heart. In other words, until the cycles build in you a greater commitment to your own happiness, fake it. Rearrange your schedule as if you were doing it for a deserving friend who is overworked and undergratified. Analyze your lifestyle, then take nips and tucks at it until you can stand back and say, "That is a nurturing, rewarding lifestyle!"

After the nurturing cycle, move on to discovering the limits cycle.

After you begin using the nurturing cycle, it is important to move right along to the cure of Effective Limits. Using the two cures together improves the strength of your nurturing considerably. Limits have a containing, soothing effect on the more intense feelings that arise. And in a sense, the limits cycle "grows us up" so that we can deal more effectively with life's realities while still honoring our deepest feelings.

It is the balance between the nurturing and limits cycles that gives your weight solution a sturdy foundation on which to rest.

Cure 2. Effective Limits

With the nurturing cure becoming part of your inner life, you are becoming more skilled at digging down deep to reach your true feelings. But the raw feelings that surface as you use the nurturing cycle are apt to be intense. Acting immediately on some of them can hurt us.

"I'm angry that I can't eat whatever I want" can lead to a major binge.

"I hate to exercise" can result in too many evenings in the easy chair.

Cure 2. Effective Limits

The strength to follow through.

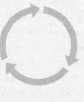

3. Essential Pain

1. Reasonable Expectations

2. Positive, Powerful Thoughts

The nurturing cycle alone can bring us back into balance with some of the feelings that arise—tired so we need sleep, hungry so we need food and lonely so we need a hug. However, other feelings must be processed through the limits cycle so that they will not harm us but, in fact, serve us well.

The diver who brings up abalone from the ocean floor must wash away sand and grit before savoring the abalone's flesh. That cleaning and tending is the role of the limits cycle. It's the combination of diving and cleaning—that is, nurturing and limits—that brings us the sweetest rewards.

The limits cycle gives us more power, more success.

Most people who use the method sink into the comfort and validation of the nurturing cycle . . . and sigh. I certainly did because life improved when I began to honor my feelings and needs. Yet soon after we have relaxed into nurturing ourselves more effectively, the value of the limits cycle becomes so apparent that it nearly glows. We can see clearly that we need *more*. We need the protection, strength and energy that effective limits can bring. As it turns out, limits are every bit as nurturing as . . . nurturing.

This is the cycle of empowerment. It's the way we "grow ourselves up" because it allows us to cut through procrastination, halt apathy and take action. We become realistic in what we expect of ourselves, others and life.

All these natural fallouts of the limits cycle not only make life better, but have a profound effect on our weight. Our resistance to eating healthfully and exercising regularly melts away. We're surprised to find ourselves going to the gym without dragging our feet. We order a salad without feeling deprived. Something profound has changed—our limits are effective.

In a moment, I'll guide you through each part of this powerful cycle: reasonable expectations; positive, powerful thinking; and facing the essential pain. As you consider this information, relax. You will not have to *force* yourself to do this. Just pick up whatever parts of the cycle excite you, and chances are you'll find yourself asking these questions unconsciously. This method is *easy* because *the tools are so powerful* that you don't need to use them

Taming Our Feelings and Gaining Control:
The Limits Cycle

"I'm angry that I can't eat whatever I want."

Expectations: Are my expectations reasonable?
No, few people can eat whatever they want. What
is reasonable? To lose weight, I have to make
some concessions.

Thinking: What am I saying to myself? That I'll
be miserable if I can't eat whatever I want. Is
that positive and powerful? No. What would be?
"There are lots of healthy foods you enjoy. You
can handle it. You won't fall apart."

Essential Pain: What is the essential pain?
That I can't lose weight unless I am willing to eat
healthier. What feelings does that bring up?
Anger. Sadness. Fear. Do the feelings fade? Yes,
they're beginning to. Can I follow through now
with eating healthier? Yes.

perfectly. Use the cycle in any way that you can; then watch for
the benefits that will come your way.

But first see for yourself how the limits cycle works in giving
us the power we need to tame the common and intense feelings
that come up as we try to lose weight: *resenting that we can't eat
whatever we want* and *hating to exercise.*

Taming Our Feelings and Gaining Control: *The Limits Cycle*

"I hate to exercise."

Expectations: What do I expect? To lose weight without exercising. Is that reasonable? No. I do have to exercise if I want to lose weight and feel my best. It would be a harsh expectation to exercise an hour per day. What is reasonable? I could walk a half hour per day.

Thinking: What am I saying to myself? "Exercise is painful and boring." Is that powerful and positive? No. What would be? "I feel better when I exercise. It's hard getting started, but then I enjoy it."

Essential Pain: What is the essential pain? That I can't sit all the time. I must exercise sometimes when I don't feel like it. What feelings does that bring up? Anger. Self-pity. Do the feelings fade? They are beginning to. Can I follow through now with exercising? Yes. It won't be so bad.

The Limits Cycle, Part 1
Are my expectations reasonable?

"How do I know what I expect of myself? I haven't even thought about it!"

"What is a reasonable expectation? How on earth would I know?"

For most of us, bringing our expectations to a conscious level is a major revelation. We may have been asked a thousand times while growing up if our shoes were tied or our teeth were brushed. But how often were we asked what we expected? The answer for most of us is *probably never.* If the expectations that were set for us in our early years were off target—that is, either too high or too low—how will we know what's reasonable to expect of ourselves or others?

"How should I know what I expect of myself?"

According to Kevin, "There was a lot of confusion in my home when I was growing up, so that I didn't know what to expect from minute to minute. My stepfather always had harsh expectations of me. He was downright mean. My mom would periodically come to my rescue, but only when she wasn't depressed. I was focused on reacting to what was going on outside of me and didn't have any idea what was reasonable to expect from them or myself."

This part of the limits cycle stimulates us to be aware of our thoughts, both conscious expectations and the unconscious ones that govern our actions. As you begin asking yourself the questions *What are my expectations?* and *Are they reasonable?* you're likely to find out more about yourself than you ever imagined. Often, when I become aware of one of my absolutely impossible and completely unstated expectations, I laugh or moan to myself, "How could I expect *that*? That's nowhere near *reasonable!*"

High expectations at work; low ones at home

Kevin's expectations were typical—"I walk into a restaurant. I'm trying to lose weight but I go in there anyway, ready to eat whatever they serve up that appeals to me. It crosses my mind to limit what I eat, but it never happens. Everything's just too tempting. Then I'm disappointed when I don't lose weight. What I discovered was that on some completely irrational level, I actually expected to lose weight while eating whatever I wanted to eat.

"Of course those expectations were not at all reasonable, but until I used the limits cycle, I never even knew what I expected, let alone that those expectations did not jibe at all with reality. Here I had always thought of myself as someone who was pretty hard on himself. But that wasn't the case at all. I expect too much of myself at work and too little of myself at home. I used overworking as a unconscious excuse to expect almost nothing of myself when it comes to eating, or I should say, overeating."

Kevin had two modes of limits: overly high ones like those his stepfather had for him and overly low ones like his mother's. This pattern of facing two extremes of expectations, without any middle ground, is not only common but typically reflects the emotional interplay between parents. Let me step back and explain that.

In many unhappy marriages, one parent, typically the mother, becomes overly indulgent and permissive with the child. In so doing, the mother reaps emotional rewards she isn't getting from her adult relationship.

The other parent, typically the father, who already feels dissatisfied and emotionally left out, feels further pushed away by this intensely close mother-child relationship. He's also upset about the effect of his wife's indulgence on the child and overcompensates by being hard on the child, expecting too much.

As a consequence, the child grows up knowing two kinds of expectations: those that are too high and those that are too low.

This same pattern operates *within* the permissive parent as well. It's irritating to live with indulged children because they develop so many annoying habits. Their rooms are a mess, their pets go unfed, and their homework is misplaced. The parent feels frustrated with the behavior but doesn't express the annoyance—and the child becomes further entrenched in irritating behaviors. Increasingly, the parent experiences subtle feelings of rejection toward the ill-behaved child, which in turn evoke a sense of guilt. That rejection is often so disturbing to parents that they mask it by further indulging the child, and parent and child grow more emotionally distant.

The parents' unexpressed anger slowly builds until frustrations are vented and harsh words fly. They then feel guilty for their sharp tongues, and a new cycle of indulgence and aloofness begins. The flip side of indulgence is often persecution, so even children with seemingly permissive parents are exposed to both harsh and easy limits. Knowing only the extremes of expectations, they lack balance.

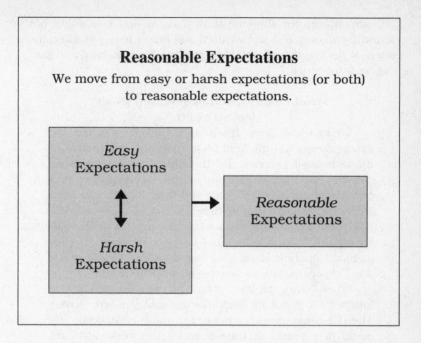

Reasonable Expectations

We move from easy or harsh expectations (or both) to reasonable expectations.

Easy
Expectations

↕

Harsh
Expectations

Reasonable
Expectations

In our groups, each participant takes a situation that is upsetting them—something that puts them off balance—and restores their inner balance by using the nurturing and limits cycle out loud in the group. The participants listening learn as much as the person speaking because in these patterns we are all the same.

What continues to amaze me is the predictable change in a person's face when they take out the tool of the limits cycle from their satchel of the six cures and make the small adjustment in their expectation so it is reasonable.

The look is like flipping a light switch—a flood of relief and often a laugh. The unconscious expectation that set them up to be stressed out, miserable and frantic was brought to a conscious level. The light switch flipped, the expectation became reasonable, and a sense of relief and relaxation washed over them.

Setting ourselves on this winning path requires surprisingly little of us. We need only be willing to ask ourselves the question "Is my expectation reasonable?" and then make a few minor adjustments in our thinking until it is. At first you might not know the answer, but rest assured that before long you'll become adept at finding the midpoint between pushing too hard and easing back too much.

"What I was expecting of myself wasn't logical at all."

When I met Gary, his main complaint was not his extra pounds but his total frustration at being unable to make himself exercise. He thought it was because he couldn't find the time. He had a full-time computer job, a hair-trimming job on the side and three kids to take care of. He rarely had a minute to himself.

I began by asking Gary what he expected of himself. He replied, "I don't know what I expect. However, if I look at how I operate, it seems I expect to lose weight and I don't expect to have to exercise in order to do it."

When Gary realized what he was expecting, he laughed. "I guess my logic doesn't make much sense." Then he came up with a more reasonable expectation: he could play tennis at least once on the weekends, and either get to the gym at work on his lunch break or play ball with his children on the other days.

Most people who begin using this cure worry that they won't be able to determine what's reasonable. Certainly such a worry makes sense because what's reasonable is highly subjective and quite variable.

But most people are like Gary. All they have to do is listen to themselves and make themselves aware of their own unspoken expectations. They can then see that their expectations are not reasonable. On the other hand, it's OK to be stumped over what is reasonable to expect.

Our challenge is not to be *right* about what makes an expectation reasonable, but to keep asking the question. Over time your expectations will slowly become more and more reasonable. As a result, you will be better able to achieve success without harming yourself.

Once you have shifted to a reasonable expectation, you have done most of the work involved in taming your feelings and enhancing your control. Using effective thinking and facing the essential pain will take you the rest of the way.

The Limits Cycle, Part 2
Are my thoughts positive and powerful?

Once your expectations are reasonable, the challenge is to meet them. Yet how do we do that? Aren't we all vulnerable to putting things off, getting stalled in a project or simply dropping the ball when other priorities arise?

Yes, of course we are, but that's not due to a character defect or a genetic flaw. In part, what gets in our way—whether our expectation is to lose a pound a week or to get up early each day for a walk—are our own thoughts. Often they are neither positive nor powerful.

> "I get all charged up to exercise, put on my running shorts and look at my legs. Do those look like the legs of an athlete? No. Forget it, and I take off the running shorts, slip into my jeans and turn on the tube."

> "I swear off sweets and then somebody brings doughnuts or cake into the office and I say to myself, 'What's the use? I can't change the world. I might as well have some of it, everybody else does.'"

Let's take those two scenarios and change them in only one way—that is, to make the voluntary, conscious thoughts of the people involved positive and powerful:

> "I get all charged up to exercise, put on my running shorts and look at my legs. My legs are getting stronger. Each time I go for a run I will be that much closer to having strong, fit legs. Maybe I'll run a little farther today."

> "I swear off sweets and then somebody brings doughnuts or cake into the office and I say to myself,'Why would I want to put greasy, sugary doughnuts in my body? These people can eat whatever they want, but I'm not eating that kind of food much these days. I think I'll get a cup of coffee and enjoy some conversation with them. Just because I'm around other people who eat in an unhealthy way doesn't mean I have to.'"

Positive, Powerful Thinking

Positive

Things will work out.

I can handle the situation.

It won't always be this way.

Something good will come from this.

I don't have to be perfect to be wonderful.

I will do the best I can and that is enough.

Powerful

I have power.

I always have at least three choices.

I have some control over this.

My feelings matter.

I can focus on now, not on the past or future.

Nothing is all black or all white.

The wise practice of showering yourself with positive, powerful thoughts

This adjustment in thinking triggers a tremendous differ-ence in emotions and actions! Just jumping from negative, powerless thinking to positive, powerful thinking saved one person from an evening on the couch watching television and another from eating doughnuts that were neither wanted nor needed.

Switching our thoughts from ineffective ones to effective ones has been a centerpiece of various mood and weight therapies for many years. Often referred to as cognitive therapy, this technique was developed by psychologist Aaron Beck, who in the early 1970's proposed that negative, powerless thinking actually causes depression and sets the stage for apathy and poor follow-through. Since then, it has been proved that changing thought patterns is a remarkably effective way to prompt changes in mood and behavior.

Noticing our thoughts and then double-checking that they are effective is a great boost for those caught in the quagmire of perfectionistic, judgmental, negative and black-and-white (all-or-nothing) thinking—all patterns common in people with weight issues. What's more, effective thoughts bring us back to the present, where our power lies, and away from excessively pondering the past or future.

Positive, powerful thoughts can prevent unnecessary lows.

Why is effective thinking so important? Because it is *difficult* to follow through. We *need* all the positive, powerful thoughts we can get—so we go for a walk when the chair beckons or take two cookies, not six, from the cookie bag. That's why responsive parents shower their children with the sincere praise and empowering talk that we are now learning to give ourselves.

What's more, positive, powerful thoughts are what keep us in the realm of balanced feelings and out of the terrain of false highs, unnecessary lows and numbness. Staying out of that terrain is essential to a weight solution because it is in that treacherous emotional territory that food abuse most often occurs.

Preventing an unnecessary low triggered by the scale.

Kristen suffered from perfectionism about her weight, which was her reason for using the method. When she joined our group she had been weighing herself twice a day and had a predictable pattern: when the number on the scale nudged upward, her mood took a roller-coaster ride downward into depression and she began alternating between restricting food and binge eating. Her thoughts about food and weight were not only obsessive, but terribly negative and destructive.

On the day of our group session, Kristen found that she had gained two pounds since the day before and had the familiar feelings that set off her cycles of obsessing about food and weight. However, this time—when the panic hit—she journeyed inside and used the limits cycle.

"I knew I couldn't change the situation—the scale wasn't lying. What I could do was use the limits cycle and see if that would help," she explained to the group.

"I checked my expectations. I have to laugh, but the truth is that I expected my weight to stay the same day to day. Is that reasonable? No. All sorts of things change it. I had pizza twice in the last three days and the salt alone could have made me gain weight. What would be reasonable? I don't know . . . to keep within a range of . . . five pounds.

Her face brightened and relaxed, but she wasn't done. Next Kristen checked her thinking.

"What am I saying to myself? Horrible things. I wouldn't talk to anybody the way I talk to myself. I was saying: *That's just the beginning. You're going to gain even more. You're out of control and you always have been.* *"What could I say to myself that would be positive and powerful? Weight is not the most important thing in life. It's normal for people's weight to fluctuate. Just because my weight changes doesn't mean I'm out of control."*

After intentionally switching her thoughts to powerful, positive ones, Kristen was back in balance. She wasn't depressed, and was able to divert herself from her familiar pattern of weight and food preoccupation.

These small adjustments in Kristen's thinking were *that* powerful, primarily because the gateway between thoughts and feelings is wide open. Our negative, powerless thoughts lead to mood changes, and our emotional roller coasters affect our thoughts. It's only when we have the tools to straighten out our thinking—that is, the limits cycle—and to be aware of our feelings—that is, the nurturing cycle—that emotional balance is likely to prevail.

It's a relief to know that the voice inside can be changed.

When Kristen recognized her thoughts, she was appalled and became indignant. She decided that the negative, powerless voice inside her had to be changed. She had so much in her life that was going well that she couldn't put up with that inner voice—which she had acquired from her mother—chipping away at her energy and leaving her drained and unhappy. Kristen didn't want to live with such an enemy inside—one that reacted to every flaw or mistake she made with judgments, criticism and negativity.

Like the rest of us, Kristen's thought style was learned and had nothing to do with her intelligence, morality, good looks or personal style. Recognizing that fact—that her thought pattern was a *choice*—changed things for Kristen. She felt *responsible* for the thought patterns because she could choose whether to keep on using her mother's critical inner voice or to *un*learn it.

If ineffective thoughts are so damaging and unpleasant, why don't we all naturally shift to positive, powerful thinking? How is choosing a positive thought pattern any different from choosing a warm cozy bed instead of a night out in the cold?

The reason is inertia, the tendency to continue familiar patterns. Interestingly, inertia and apathy are signs of ineffective nurturing and limits. Listen to what we say to ourselves:

- Everyone else does it, so why shouldn't I?

- I've always done it, so why change now?

This is *numbness.* It dampens the spirit and it kills. We stay with patterns that harm us, and despite our intelligence and sophistication in other arenas, we aren't even aware that we are doing it.

Fortunately, the nurturing cycle wakes us up to ourselves and the limits cycle separates us from the past and others. Together they stimulate us to move out of inertia and apathy and begin aggressively boycotting ineffective thinking.

Yet there is another reason that negative, powerless thoughts persist—one that is far more seductive. It is the unconscious pleasure they give in guiding us back below the separation of the generations line into the comfortable role of the child. There we can wallow in self-pity, depression, rebellion or hostility. Oddly enough, there is a certain pleasure in being down there feeling as awful as we want to feel.

I enjoy this role too. If my mind settles into a pattern of negative thinking, before long I'll find comfort in self-pity. Sure, I could snap out of my blue mood by showering myself with positive, powerful thoughts, and often I do just that. Other times, I don't.

Instead I muse to myself, "Sometimes I need to feel depressed and powerless. That's just part of me and that's good enough. It's OK not to do it *right* all the time and I'm enjoying this for now."

Inadvertently, by showing compassion toward that childish side of me, I often begin to feel better! Why? Because unintentionally I've talked to myself in a positive and powerful voice—full of acceptance, compassion and humor. Without my awareness, I've returned to the adult role and regained my inner balance.

What thought style will you use—positive and powerful or negative and powerless?

The Limits Cycle, Part 3
What is the essential pain?

The last part of the limits cycle is to feel the unavoidable pain of a situation and allow that feeling to wash over you. You can tolerate the discomfort because you know that it will fade, and when it does, that you will have the energy you needed all along to follow through.

Once you become skilled in accepting life's essential pain, you will need neither willpower nor true grit to take actions that bring you the success you want. Even those things you don't particularly enjoy doing—like scrubbing out pots, finding something, *anything*, to wear in the morning or visiting your mother-in-law—become far less troublesome. The deeper challenges of life—the risk of intimacy, the worry about health and insecurity about money—stop controlling your thoughts and running your life.

> Kristen reacted to her newfound skill in accepting essential pain: "The more I get used to accepting the essential pain of life, the more resilient I'm becoming. Even the worst thing—getting fatter, losing my job or coming down with a terrible disease—is not that bad. I've given myself far more pain trying to protect myself from facing the worst thing. The constant dieting, the constant worry are far worse than facing and getting past the essential pain."

Facing essential pain is a discrete skill that is at the heart of your weight solution. The best way to understand it is to dive in and try it. If you're willing, try facing some essential pain right now. Do it, if you can, with an attitude of curiosity—as if you're interested to see how you will react to this reality. You'll probably find that the feelings are intense, but they will go away, and you will *not* fall apart forever.

Choose one of these thoughts—or another one if you prefer—and say it to yourself. State that truth several times. Then watch your feelings—such as anger, sadness, fear, guilt—arise within you:

- My dreams may not come true.

- I'm not perfect.

- I don't have complete control.

Now watch your feelings—notice their intensity. Chances are they are rising up and if you can stay with your feelings rather than opting out of them by thinking, numbing or distracting yourself—they will continue to rise. It won't feel good, but those feelings won't increase forever. After a time, your feelings will subside, the way a bell-shaped curve falls back to baseline.

If you were able to do that—think the thought, feel the feelings and let them fade—you will now notice a huge sense of relief come over you and a big charge of energy. This is the gift of the limits cycle. If you weren't able to do it, that's fine too. You will become proficient at it in time.

It's just a skill, like riding a bike or mowing the lawn.

What surprised me most about facing the essential pain was that it became easier with practice. This certainly doesn't mean that it is easy.

As you use the limits cycle, you won't necessarily come to savor your essential pain the way you would your lover's touch or your child's smile. But you'll find that the pain becomes less grinding and frightening and more ordinary—like straightening the bed after a night of sleep or picking up your child's dirty clothes off the floor. It's simply part of the maintenance of life.

The instant payoff of essential pain: inner balance

The best reason to face essential pain is that it feels *so good* when it's over. In fact, once the feelings fade there's an almost instantaneous payoff. Instead of feeling stuck, conflicted, aggravated or depressed, you feel . . . balanced—ready to move forward and take action, whether that be talking to the boss, working out a schedule change or going for a walk.

> "I had already written off the evening. I was depressed and lonely and I knew I was going to eat. The essential pain I faced was that I am alone right now. There was no one here to support me but me. Once the sadness of that realization faded, my appetite vanished. Why overeat? That was not a solution. I felt incredibly proud that I didn't numb myself with food that evening."

> "I faced the essential pain that if I wanted to have a better relationship with my husband, I'd have to be willing to meet him halfway, and I felt tremendously relieved. I made that concession, and I found myself giving to him more. That was the turning point in our relationship."

The process is simple.

Gliding through your essential pain is a bit like taking out a splinter. A little courage is needed to pull out the splinter. But if you don't pull it out, you risk infection and further pain. Facing your essential pain requires being willing to experience some discomfort without falling apart, then reaping the rewards. *This is something you can do.*

Some people like to express their essential pain; others like to contain it and be alone with their distress. One close friend holes himself away when upset; another calls me hourly. Yet the internal process is the same. We must feel it and release it.

The most rewarding kinds of essential pain

There are daily sources of essential pain: turning off the alarm, rude salespeople and work deadlines. These are the nuts and bolts of daily life. In addition, there are the existential hurts

Gliding Through Your Essential Pain

1. State it.
State what the essential pain is, that is, the
reality you must face in order to follow through.
"I am not perfect."
"I can't control what will happen."

2. Feel it.
Hearing that fact brings up feelings.
Notice those feelings.
"That makes me sad."
"I feel angry and afraid."

3. Avoid thoughts.
Thoughts block your feelings before they have
been fully felt. You lose the opportunity to
strengthen yourself.
"What am I feeling?"
"Stay with the feeling."

4. Watch the feeling fade.
The feelings will rise, then subside. Watch them
leave you and notice how much stronger you feel.

5. Follow through.
Take action and follow through successfully with the
reasonable expectation you set for yourself.

of chronic anxiety, isolation of the self, spiritual yearnings and the
certainty of death.

But by far the most difficult essential pain for many of us is that
required for intimacy. Human intimacy is always intense, sometimes fragile and fleeting and other times strong and enduring.

As Father Flynn, a Paulist father with the Newman Center at Berkeley, told me, the intimate moment between humans on earth is a microcosm of the unity between the human and the divine. It can also be exceedingly dangerous. According to David Schnarck, a noted family therapist, the desiring of another and the concommitant drive to maintain that desire *demand* that our nurturing and limits skills be more than fledgling—they must be completely intact. Without those skills pumping at full speed, according to Schnarck, love wanes and desire departs.

Clearly, *mature love is not for kids.* It requires us to grow up, to be able to affirm and nurture ourselves yet be willing to risk abandonment or surrender. No wonder so many of us go to the refrigerator instead of to the arena of human closeness.

The sweetness of intimacy . . .

So if food is love and we must stop needing food so much if we are to solve a weight problem, then it's time to bring on the love. Out goes the isolation. In comes the warmth, closeness, sensuality and comfort on which we can thrive: intimacy.

But there's also the moment when intimacy fails. Perhaps we aren't compatible with that person after all, or we don't have luck on our side, or we've not *both* mastered the six cures. Intimate relationships can be a minefield of power struggles, rejection, manipulation, withdrawal and numbness.

Intimacy—the ripest fruit of life—is to be found at the top of the tree. Experiencing it requires us to stretch—a stretch that involves facing the essential pain involved in closeness.

. . . and the essential pain of closeness

Several years ago when the university experienced a series of violent crimes on campus during daylight hours, I signed up for self-defense classes. But before the first class session, I read a study that impressed me so much I canceled my enrollment.

The study revealed that taking self-defense classes didn't always affect people's reactions to potential perpetrators. Why? Because certain individuals couldn't bring themselves to hurt their aggressors. In other words, they could not face the essential

The Essential Pain of Intimacy

- I must be present in the current moment.
- I must allow myself to be exposed.
- I must acknowledge that both of us have needs.
- I must be willing to give and to receive.
- I must risk the possibility of rejection or surrender.

pain involved in using their self-defense skills. I saw myself in that study. I knew that I would be one of those who screamed ineffectually rather than violently attacking the aggressor.

In a similar way, couples trying to improve their relationships often focus on communication skills, which can be helpful. But they probably won't use those skills unless they have faced the essential pain of intimacy.

Which of these sources of essential pain are you willing to feel and let fade?

Once we have faced these sources of essential pain, we can get on with the business of enhancing the communication skills we need for intimacy:

- Opening up and sharing yourself—that is, *putting out the line*
- Receiving what another gives with gratitude—that is, *savoring the tender morsel*

Not only do these skills help us achieve an intimate connection, but using them also heals childhood wounds. One or the other of these two skills puts us right back into feeling the vulnerability we felt as children. And if we feel as vulnerable as we did back then, but overcome it, the wound from the past begins to mend. The specific skill that will provide the greatest rewards for your own healing typically depends on the thickness of the boundaries you've developed.

Putting out the line

If your boundaries tend to be thick, your challenge will be to open up and express your feelings and needs. Most people would do this if they knew a way to make opening up safer. The nurturing cycle will help. Most participants in groups use it as a formula for opening up. It keeps them out of their usual patterns of talking about thoughts, staying aloof or entering into arguments that are nothing more than power struggles.

You already know how to do it. Putting out the line is just saying aloud your answers to the questions of the nurturing cycle. Just using those words *"I feel . . . ," "I need . . ."* and *"Would you please . . ."* is remarkably effective. Try it and see for yourself!

Receiving a tender morsel

If your boundaries are relatively thin, your challenge will be to receive from another and to appreciate what you receive. Instead of taking a tidbit and running away, feel the caring it was sent with. Express your appreciation for the gift and the giver.

This can be frightening and feel invasive. To receive from

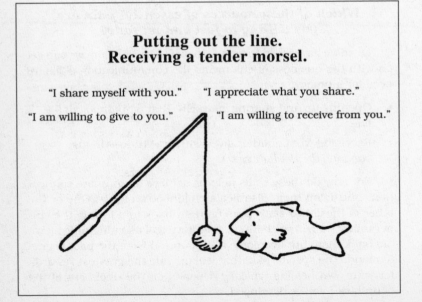

Putting out the line.
Receiving a tender morsel.

"I share myself with you."   "I appreciate what you share."

"I am willing to give to you."   "I am willing to receive from you."

The Skills of Intimacy

If our boundaries are thick, we need to practice
putting out the line:
*Opening up enough to share who we are, and
being willing to give to another.*

If our boundaries are thin, we need to practice
receiving the tender morsel:
*Closing ourselves enough to experience ourselves
and accept and value what another person
has shared or given.*

another requires you to feel. It is scary to allow a gift to seep into your very being, where even you may not want to go. It would be far easier to treat the tender morsel as if it were meaningless and without value. But the opportunity for intimacy would be lost.

Creating intimacy is a skill.

Compare the difference for yourself. Here is the standard quarrel that group members say they experience with their partners. These brief interchanges often vex them to the point of running to the refrigerator, losing interest in lovemaking or going on strike on the couch. First let's listen in on the way it begins.

No line. No tender morsels.

"I can't stand what's happening. You've got to stop it!"
"I won't talk to you. I have nothing to say."
"You'll never change."
"You bet I won't!"

Now watch what happens when one person is open and giving and the other appreciates and receives.

Putting out the line and receiving a tender morsel

"I feel sad and worried about what is happening. I *need* to talk with you about it so we can come up with some ideas about how to change things. *Would you please* take some time to talk with me about it?"

"I *understand* that you are upset about it. I *appreciate* that you brought it up. I know it wasn't easy for you. Yes, let's talk about it now."

Both people got what they wanted. Cooperation instead of a control struggle. A chance that they will solve the problem. And, perhaps most important, rather than a moment of detachment, a time of closeness and healing.

Since a kernel of intimacy can be present in any interaction between two people, you'll probably begin noticing the dynamic of putting out the line and taking the tender morsel in all your encounters with others. Do *you* put out the line and receive the tender morsel? Do *they*?

Here is an example.

Recently, at the end of a Solution group meeting, one woman, Robin, said she'd have to stop coming to the sessions. She had lost her ride and no buses were available. According to Robin, she had no choice but to quit.

Candace responded, "I'll drive you."

Robin said, "OK," and changed the subject to ask about the next session.

There it was. Candace had an opportunity to open up and convey in words, as well as actions, that she cared about Robin. She could have put out the line, but she didn't. Robin, for her part, passed up a chance to show gratitude and appreciation for Candace's generous offer, the tender morsel she had been offered.

Their blocks in intimacy skills were perfectly predictable.

Both of these patterns were completely understandable. Because Robin's mother and father were seriously involved in politics and their careers, Robin had been the mother to her four younger siblings. Thus she was comfortable with giving, but not at all used to receiving. It was hard to trust that someone would give to her.

On a more subtle level, if Robin acknowledged the emotional acceptance that Candace's offer represented, she risked feeling and exposing her inner emptiness. It was much safer to deny her own needs and to reject the generosity. Yet only through receiving could Robin effectively chip away at her emotional armor, her thick boundaries, and allow some intimacy to seep in.

Candace was raised by a single mother who was overprotective and pampered her only child every way she could. Since her mother had given endlessly to her, taking was second nature to Candace. It was giving to others that felt somewhat odd and definitely frightening to her. Would she know how much to give and when to stop? Would her gift be valued? Would she surrender herself in the process, not knowing when to stop giving? However, in learning to give, Candace took her largest step toward reaping the rewards of intimacy.

In our group we all paused. We could all see in our own relationships the dynamic Candace and Robin were experiencing. On the board I drew a picture of the line with the morsel and the fish, saying that for an intimate connection to occur, both people must be able to put out the line and receive the tender morsel. Often it seems we are much better at one than the other. Robin and Candace understood at once.

Once they understood the pattern, the changes began.

Robin volunteered, "That was a generous offer Candace made, and I didn't even acknowledge it. I didn't even act like I appreciated what she was offering to do for me."

Candace looked surprised. "I didn't even notice that you didn't acknowledge me."

It may seem that I'm splitting hairs because clearly Candace did make an offer and Robin did take her up on it. However, by using the tools of the method what started as an empty exchange between these two women became a fulfilling friendship.

There was a potential danger, however. Their opposite

vulnerabilities had made them comfortable with their original exchange, which would be fine for the short run but would lead to certain disappointment as the relationship continued.

Robin was comfortable giving. It was her knee-jerk reaction to another person's needs, an external solution. When she gave, she was not aware of the strength, wisdom and goodness within herself, so she gave without emotion and even without reason. Often she gave far too much, then cut off friendships because others were "ungrateful" or "selfish."

By the same token, Candace was used to accepting favors or good deeds without also accepting the emotional gift and without understanding what it required of the other person to give to her. Like Robin, Candace was not connected to her inner strength, wisdom and goodness. She was therefore vulnerable to taking in excess, eventually resulting in the other person feeling used and unappreciated and going away—much to her surprise and hurt.

Facing the essential pain opened the door to intimacy.

Yet if both women were willing to face the essential pain of intimacy and begin to use these intimacy skills, their friendship wouldn't end in disaster. It could instead slowly evolve and deepen into a balanced and fulfilling connection.

Robin turned to Candace. "I feel embarrassed about not acknowledging you for offering to do so much for me. It's hard for me to receive. The essential pain I must face and let fade is that I have needs—I can't do everything myself. And that you might judge me and reject me for being so needy."

Candace paused. "You didn't need to acknowledge me giving you the ride, because I didn't act as if I were offering you anything but a ride. What I didn't say was that I have enjoyed knowing you in the group and I want to continue to spend time with you. It's hard for me to accept the essential pain that if I put out the line and tell you these things, you might not value what I'm giving you. It's hard for me to take that risk."

The rest of the group was hushed for a moment, then exploded in applause, for each of us could see herself in what Robin and Candace had so bravely said. That was the beginning of a vital friendship that would never have occurred if they had not faced the essential pain of intimacy and ventured out to more vulnerable positions.

What this valiant effort required was that each woman journey inside herself, regain her inner balance, and then take the risk of opening up and giving, or of receiving with gratitude. They had each experienced using a skill that they could transfer to many relationships to enhance the intimacy in their lives. Interestingly, this session was a turning point in both women's weight: they began to lose pounds with little conscious effort.

The essential pain of your weight solution . . .

Please pause for a moment and use the checklist on the next page to face, feel and let fade the essential pain of losing weight.

Read each statement slowly. Notice the feelings that arise in you and watch them fade. This is a time to face the essential pain of weight loss and to let those feelings fade away.

Enough is enough. Change the outside, not the inside.

Now your expectations are more reasonable—neither too high nor too low—and you can go forward expecting neither too much nor too little of yourself and life. In essence you know your limits and have the skill to set them. It is the perfect time to conduct lifestyle surgery, to make basic, enduring changes in your life.

Where you move your scalpel, and how deep or wide the cut, is completely individual. You are an adult. You know what you can and can't take anymore. You recognize what does and doesn't work for you.

By making a conceptual decision to change something, you give your decision staying power. You can better protect yourself day to day and will no longer be burdened with situations that do not foster your health and happiness.

The Strength to Follow Through

In order to solve my weight problem, I am willing to accept the essential pain that I must:

_____ put limits on my eating.

_____ exercise daily, even at times when I don't feel like it.

_____ journey inside myself throughout the day.

_____ nurture myself in ways other than overeating.

_____ set more reasonable expectations for myself.

_____ feel compassionate and accepting toward my body and myself.

_____ take good care of my health.

_____ engage in activities that are meaningful to me.

_____ take time to restore my mind, body and soul.

Stand back from your life for a few minutes and ask yourself, "What limits must I set so that I will be happier and healthier?"

Others have answered this question and done lifestyle surgery in the following ways:

"I must set limits on my work. I'm going to leave the office at 6:00 P.M."

"I'm not going to have my parents as house guests anymore. It's just too difficult."

"I can't tolerate having credit cards in my pocket. I'm cutting them up."

"My children are wonderful, but I need a break for myself. One evening a week I'm getting a sitter."

"I can't wait for dinner at 8:00 anymore. I'll eat by myself earlier."

"This is a dead-end job. I must start job hunting."

"I can't ignore my appearance anymore. I'm going to budget myself some clothes money."

"Drinking is a problem for me. I'm going to stop it cold turkey."

You now have the power to soothe yourself from within.

No one can take from you your ability to journey inside, to draw on the nurturing and limits cycles and, if need be, the other cycles to bring yourself back to emotional balance. You will never be alone, because you can always connect with your inherent strength, wisdom and goodness. What's more, mastering the remainder of the cures will become far easier for you because the remaining cures are built on the foundation of nurturing and limits.

For more ideas about how to use the cycles together to balance both thoughts and feelings, read the examples on the next few pages, taken from the words of participants in the program at the university.

Then go on to the next step, which is to acquaint yourself with the cycles that bring balance to the body: Body Pride and Good Health.

A Few Journeys through the Mind Cycles

The cycles are very adaptable. Most likely you'll use them in the order presented, beginning with nurturing, then going on to limits, over and over again if need be, until you are back in balance. However, sometimes you may find that starting with the limits cycle or asking yourself only some of the six questions of these cures is as rewarding. The idea is to feel perfectly comfortable using the tools of the method in any way that responds to your inner needs and to your personal preferences.

Situation No. 1: Eating binges

Marsha, the office supervisor who was dealing with the needs of a dying husband and a beloved mother with Alzheimer's, had almost mastered the method but continued to experience periodic eating binges that devastated her.

If she binged once, she would continue for the entire weekend. By the time she returned to work on Monday, she was bloated, miserable and depressed. Marsha was able to regain her inner balance and cut down considerably on her binge eating by using the cycles.

The Nurturing Cycle

I feel . . . angry at myself, stupid for eating again and guilty that I can't stop.

I need . . . to forgive myself, get some exercise and enjoy the rest of my day.

Would you please . . . can do this myself.

The Limits Cycle

I expect . . . that I won't ever binge again. That's not reasonable. What is? That I may binge before my period or when I haven't taken enough time to restore myself.

I think . . . that I should be perfect. That isn't helping. What would be positive and powerful? That I will do the best I can. Just because I binge doesn't mean I am bad or wrong. It's just a pattern that I am in the process of releasing.

The essential pain . . . is that I'm not perfect and that I may binge-eat forever. What feelings come up? Sadness (she feels the sadness) . . . but it's beginning to fade. I can go on, get some exercise and enjoy my day.

Situation No. 2: Money worries

Jack, the attorney who specialized in intellectual properties and shared a law practice with his three buddies from grammar school, was troubled not only by eating problems but also by his spending.

Just before our meeting, he had opened his mail to find a pile of bounced checks. He knew that his billing hours at work weren't increasing, but his spending was. His wife immediately blamed him for the problem, and Jack went into orbit. How dare she blame him and try to control him? He worked hard. He was entitled to spend money like everybody else.

In the next session, he regained his inner balance by using the cycles.

The Nurturing Cycle

I feel . . . embarrassed about my spending and angry at my wife for telling me I have to stop spending so much.

I need . . . to reassure myself that my needs will be met, even if I don't spend as much money. I can survive with having less. I need my wife to stop blaming me. She doesn't work full time, and she also overspends.

Would you please . . . stop speaking to me in a blaming tone when we discuss money. I know it is difficult for you too, but would you please meet with me to discuss what we can both do to make our money situation better?

The Limits Cycle

I expect . . . that I can spend as much as I want, which isn't reasonable. What is? That I have to cut back somewhat but not deny myself everything. I also expect that my wife will continue overspending and working part time, even if I make concessions to spend less.

I think . . . that I'll never get the things I want. I think my wife won't do her part. Are those thoughts helping? No. What would be more positive and powerful? It would be to say that our money situation could improve and we could cooperate in making this happen.

The essential pain . . . is that if I don't set limits on my spending I'll go bankrupt. If I do set limits on my spending, I won't have all the things I want. The essential pain is also that my wife might not cooperate. What feelings arise? Anger and fear. They're fading. I can talk with my wife and try to improve our situation.

Situation No. 3: Encountering the family

Darcy, the tall, dark-haired woman with the hearty laugh and the French café that offered country and western singing, was uncharacteristically glum at one session. When I inquired what was bothering her, she said it was her family. They were planning a family vacation with all her brothers and sisters and their kids. Nobody in the family got along, and her brother was apt to drink too much and become rude.

Moreover, Darcy longed for a child. It was difficult for her to face all the joy her siblings had received from their large broods of kids. Darcy used the cycles to bring herself back into emotional balance.

The Nurturing Cycle

I feel . . . sad that I don't have kids.

I need . . . to have kids. Or to make peace with not having them. Or to decide what my options are now for having my own kids or for adopting a child.

Would you please . . . I must start talking with friends about this. It's a sensitive issue with me and I haven't been open to discussing it with people. And I have to look into what my options are.

The Limits Cycle

I expect . . . that there won't be any good answer for me. I feel doomed to being childless. Is that reasonable? No. Actually there are many possibilities.

I think . . . that I won't have kids in my life. It will never work out for me. Is that helping? No. What could I say to myself that would be positive and powerful? That the future is not known. There is hope, and it's my job to explore what possibilities there are.

The essential pain . . . is that I may not have kids. What feelings does that bring up? Anger, frustration, sadness and guilt. I've worked through these feelings before. I know they'll fade. Actually I feel energized to find out my options now. I think I can get on with the business of dealing with this situation.

Still Darcy wasn't back in balance. Rather than letting it go, thinking, "Oh well, I feel a little better. That's good enough for me," and essentially abandoning herself, she stayed with the cycles until she regained her emotional balance.

The Nurturing Cycle

I feel . . . afraid of dealing with my family this summer. I am afraid we'll get into an argument and the vacation will be spoiled.

I need . . . to make a plan for how I will handle the situation if my brother starts drinking and making rude remarks to me.

Would you please . . . listen to me while I try to figure out what I will do?

The Limits Cycle

I expect . . . that he will be nasty and crude. Is that reasonable? No. Sometimes he is rather personable. What else do I expect? That I can't protect myself from his remarks. Is that reasonable? No. I can remove myself from the situation or speak to him with assertion, giving him a "hamburger sandwich" that expresses my needs.

I think . . . that I am powerless against him, and that doesn't help. What would be something positive and powerful that I could say to myself? That I don't have to take his abuse and that I can protect myself. I could say that we may end up having a pleasant time together, who knows?

The essential pain . . . is that I can't control all that happens when I see my brother. It may end up being unpleasant. What feelings come up? Sadness (she feels the sadness). . . . It does fade . . . I'm not upset about seeing my family now. I feel back in balance.

Cure 3. Body Pride

We don't talk very much about food and eating around our home, but one morning last week my teenage daughter, Haley, was exasperated. "Mom, all the girls at school, even the ones with beautiful bodies, think they're fat. They're starving themselves all the time, then eating all this junk food. You should *do something* about it!"

I smiled to myself, because in the mid-1980's, when Haley was just entering kindergarten, my colleagues and I were among the first to study the prevalence of eating disorder characteristics, including distorted body image, in children. The results were

Cure 3. Body Pride

Honoring and accepting your body.

**3. Honor and
Accept**

**1. Avoid
Weightism**

2. Use Words, Not Weight

startling. Our survey of about 500 children in San Francisco showed that more than 80 percent of girls in the fourth grade exhibited at least one characteristic of eating disorders, such as binge eating, purging, restrictive eating and body image distortion. What's more, even by that very early stage of life, a sizable portion of them thought they were fat, although their weight was perfectly normal.

I reassured my daughter. "Haley, I know it's disturbing to see your friends rejecting their bodies, but their feelings aren't just about their weight. It's a matter that's far deeper. Self-image and body image are hopelessly intertwined."

Haley seemed to be listening, but was still upset.

"Your friends will reject some part of their appearance— whether it is their weight, their height or their shape—until they reach a point where they can accept themselves *on the inside*. When they accomplish that, it will be more than a skin-deep victory. In a sense, it will be a statement that they have grown up."

As I dropped Haley off at school, I thought to myself: It's a bit more complicated than that. Because body and self are intertwined, unraveling them is very difficult. What people don't like about themselves becomes projected onto some part of their body, which they then disparage. And what people dislike about their bodies becomes fodder for rejection of the self. Rejection of the body and self add to the buildup of emotional distress inside. We stop seeking comfort from within ourselves and start seeking external gratifiers in excess.

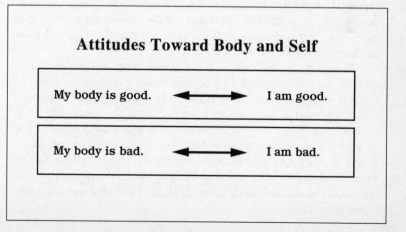

Attitudes Toward Body and Self

My body is good. ⟷ I am good.

My body is bad. ⟷ I am bad.

If body pride is so important, why don't they package it?

So there was no simple solution to Haley's worries about her friends' body shame. Body pride is a mark of maturity that is hard to attain in our culture. It is more than losing weight, buying new clothes or finding the right hair style. It is an inside job, requiring a strong foundation in the other cures plus mastery of all three parts of the body pride cycle: avoiding weightist thoughts; using words, not weight, to express yourself; and honoring and accepting your body and yourself.

Like refinishing the finest of woods . . .

The body pride cycle is unique among the cures. It is far more abstract, and its ideas require the tincture of time to become fully apparent. Just when you think you've mastered this cure, you uncover a whole new layer of understanding. Mastering the body pride cycle is not an overnight phenomenon for anyone.

Working on this cure is like refinishing the finest of woods. If you were to refinish a walnut table that your grandfather made, you'd patiently and gently strip away the layers of old finish one at a time until you got to the raw, smooth wood. Then you'd apply the thinnest of coats of new finish over and over again. As you refinish your body attitudes, you will return to this cure over and over again, each time laying down a little more body pride and a little more self-acceptance. In the end, your body pride will glow as beautifully as a family heirloom.

Even though this cure is more subtle and abstract than the rest, it's no less powerful. In fact, mastering it is often the turning point upon which a weight solution rests. So many times a person using the method appears to have cured all the causes of their weight issue, but the number on the scale stays stubbornly stuck at a level that is clearly above their body's genetic comfort zone. When that frustrating situation occurs, the missing link in the weight solution is almost always body pride. In the pages that follow I will show you exactly how to put this powerhouse of a cure to work for you.

"*Stop everything.* I won't have body pride until I'm thin."

If you insist on rejecting your body until you lose weight, I will never argue the point with you. It's an argument I can't win. I will, however, mention a few ideas that you might consider as you master this cure.

First, entertain the idea that your current weight is a blessing, not a curse. *Before you skip to the next paragraph, let me clarify.* People approach this method for a purpose. To lose weight. If it weren't for the visible presence of their weight, they would kick back and spend the time you are spending right now, not on transforming their lives, but in watching the sports channel, taking hot baths, reading the paper or chatting on the phone.

They need *every ounce* of their current body weight to catalyze their mastery of this method. Think of that weight as a minor scrape on the finger. Because of the scrape, people may reluctantly get up off the couch, walk into the bathroom, open the medicine cabinet and find not only a bandage but a transformation of their whole lives.

That *annoying scrape* was needed, just the way we need the issue of weight. Consider pulling back from hating your weight, and beginning to see it as a blessing. After all, it led you to open some doors and give yourself what you needed the most.

Body pride means gaining control, not losing it.

The second idea is as difficult to hear and as important as the first.

Many of us with weight concerns believe that if we accept our body as it is, something terrible will happen. We'll get totally out of control, our appetites will spiral upward and our bodies will become bigger and bigger.

In truth, the opposite will occur.

I saw this firsthand in the clinic at the university. A mother from the poorest section of the city brought in her overweight teenage daughter, who was glum and withdrawn. Nothing seemed to register with her; she was totally tuned out. This didn't stop her mother from hollering at her. I asked the mother to pause a moment and listen to herself. I suggested that a nurturing word might be a way to motivate her daughter to lose weight.

The mother stuck her chin out and squinted her eyes. "You're crazy. If I give in to her, she'll give into herself and then she'll be on drugs, stealing and running with the wrong kinds of boys."

Distrust and overcontrol can't heal us.

Although this mother's reaction to her daughter may sound extreme, her attitude may be the very same one you're showing right now—toward your own body!

Ultimately it's *compassion* for the self that heals, whether that compassion has philosophical, spiritual or pragmatic origins. The dynamic that had triggered a weight problem in this girl was very cold and judgmental attitudes. How could it be solved by *more* coldness and *more* judgment?

The judge in you, the negative voice, may pound the gavel and shout weightist accusations and rebukes. That judge has probably insisted that because you aren't perfect, you must be awful, that because you aren't in total control of your weight, you are powerless, and that you'll always struggle with your weight.

You can fire your own judge.

The answer is not to submit to the judge's harsh ruling, but to fire him! Throw him out on his ear! And in place of that lecturing judge welcome a compassionate guide who lays down the gavel, holds your hand and is pleased to regard you. And that guide, who knows every ounce of you inside and out, will tell you:

- "Your body is beautiful just the way it is."

- "You are wonderful because you are you."

- "You don't need to fix yourself. You are not broken."

These words are at the heart of a compassionate, loving relationship with yourself. This acceptance is so powerful that when you allow a compassionate voice to live inside you, you won't have *lost* your control, you'll have *gained* it. For inner balance and the high degree of control it offers flourish in a warm and nourishing environment, one of self-regard.

The Body Pride Cycle, Part 1
Avoiding weightist thoughts

I admit to still wincing every year when the swimsuit issue of *Sports Illustrated* arrives and I see the stampede of men lining up at magazine stands. I ask myself, "*Why couldn't I look like that? What's wrong with me, anyway?*" and, if I let my ineffective thinking go too far, I'll hear myself say, "*I'm just a failure. I'll never measure up,*" and I sink into despair.

In that situation, I've allowed weightist messages to take me to task. Usually, I'm not even aware that I've allowed those thoughts in until I experience the dreary consequence of body shame. The problem is that weightist thoughts are at once so silent and deadly, not only must we vigilantly watch for them, we must fight back and forcefully eject them from our inner lives.

Stop the hurting so the healing can begin.

Before the true healing of our body image—and self-image—can begin, we must first stop beating ourselves up with weightist thoughts.

Hurting must stop before healing can begin. Jan West, a minister who is devoted to serving the burgeoning Hispanic population in my community, has taught me well about healing. When I sought her counsel about my own difficulties in healing a serious hurt, she was quick to point out the effects of my self-judgment. Compassionately and softly she said, "Laurel, you can't expect yourself to start healing yourself until you *stop* hurting yourself. You must stop the negative, judging thoughts that punish you."

In the same way, you must stop weightist thoughts in order to open the door to the healing of your body image and your self-regard. Ridding yourself of weightist thoughts takes two internal maneuvers on your part:

Body Pride Thoughts

Avoiding our own weightism.

My body doesn't have to be perfect to be wonderful.

Bodies come in all sizes and shapes.

I honor and accept my body.

All bodies are good bodies, including mine.

Avoiding the weightism of others.

If people judge my weight, that's their problem.

Weightism is no better than racism or sexism.

Keep your weightism to yourself!

I feel sorry for them because they are weightists.

- Stop harming yourself. Substitute body pride statements for weightist statements.

- Force the weightist messages of others to bounce off you with the help of your own body pride statements and by using the nurturing and limits cycles.

Douse the hot flames of your own weightism.

Yet how do you know the weightists aren't *right?* Maybe your weight *does* mean there is something wrong with you. Maybe you *don't* measure up. Stop right there. Despite the perfectionistic, judgmental side of you, the reality is that weight prejudices are utterly groundless.

The differences between pencil-thin and more robust people are small and inconsequential, yet they've been distorted beyond reason in our culture because of two cultural obsessions: control and perfection. It's the fear in others of losing control and being imperfect that fans the flames of weightism. It is fear, not reality. For there are hundreds of studies comparing lean and overweight people and they show very small differences between the groups. What is the truth about people with weight problems?

The facts:

On the average, people with weight problems don't eat significantly more calories or burn off any fewer calories from exercise than normal-weight people.

The subtle differences in eating patterns and activity levels between overweight and lean people—overweight people eat more fat and exercise less intensely—are not moral or ethical issues.

Weight has no effect whatsoever on a person's ability to take on the important roles in life: to be a good friend, a good parent, a good worker or a good citizen.

"Weightism is all around me.
How do I protect myself?"

Essentially you use the nurturing and limits cures. Expressing anger at the discrimination helps. Determining what you need to combat weightism can't hurt, and switching your expectations and thinking so that they are on your side is an obvious winner. Last, facing the essential pain that you may always have weightist thoughts and you cannot completely control the weightism will help you move forward in reclaiming your body pride.

Let's look at some common situations we all encounter in our weightist culture and what you could say to yourself to give yourself the protection you deserve.

Situation No. 1: A Diet Soda Commercial

You are watching a television show with a friend and repeatedly see a soda commercial featuring happy, young, beautiful, skinny women and attractive, powerful, slender men.

The Nurturing Cycle

I feel . . . jealous, inadequate, angry and sad that I don't look like that.

I need . . . to stop being such a weightist. Most people don't look like that. And even those who do have their own problems.

Would you please . . . turn the channel.

The Limits Cycle

I expect . . . myself to look like them. Is that reasonable? No. They are one in a million and the rest of us aren't.

I think . . . that I look unattractive. Is that helping? No. What could I say to myself that would be positive and powerful? I look good. So what if I don't look like a Barbie or Ken doll. My appearance is unique. People like people for their insides too, and I'm funny and smart.

The essential pain . . . is that I'll never look like them or be them. What feelings come up? Some sadness. Some regret. But actually it's not that bad. I'm a happy enough person.

Situation No. 2: An Insensitive Child

You are walking down the street on a Saturday with your partner, and a little boy points at you and says loudly to his mother, "That person is so fat."

The Nurturing Cycle

I feel . . . embarrassed, angry and ashamed.

I need . . . to calm down and soothe myself. What just happened hurt.

Would you please . . . pardon me. I need to walk without talking while I calm myself down after what just happened.

The Limits Cycle

I expect . . . not to be ridiculed. Is that a reasonable expectation? No. Most people are ridiculed at some times in their lives about something.

I think . . . that the child is right. I am a fat person. Are those thoughts helping? No. What would be something positive and powerful I could say to myself? That the child is just a child and probably learned weightism from his parents. It's sad that he is already a weightist.

The essential pain . . . is that there will always be people who ridicule other people and I may be the recipient of ridicule again. That hurts. If I stay with that pain it does begin to go away. There are worse things in life. Now I feel balanced again and can enjoy the day and my partner again.

Situation No. 3: A Critical Relative

At a family party you notice a female relative looking over your body in a judgmental way. Later, that same person asks you how your diet is going and comments about how good you looked when you were thinner than you are now.

The Nurturing Cycle

I feel . . . sad that she's so weight-focused, furious that she judged me and guilty for not having lost weight.

I need . . . to get away from her judgment, either physically or by using words.

Would you please . . . not talk about my weight. It's not something I feel like discussing right now.

The Limits Cycle

I expect . . . her to stop bothering me about my weight. Is that a reasonable expectation? No, not for this relative. She's relentless. What is a reasonable expectation? That to get her to stop I'll have to avoid her or make another request that has more muscle in it, such as "Would you please drop the subject? I'd like to continue our conversation, but I don't want to if weight is the topic."

I think . . . that I am powerless, trapped with a woman who is critical. Is that helping? No. What would be positive and powerful? To say to myself that I always have choices and options. I don't need to be passive and allow myself to feel attacked.

The essential pain . . . is that I have some critical relatives that I have to see again. What feelings come up when I face that fact?

Irritation. Sadness. But it's lessening now. This is such a hassle, but I feel back in balance. I can handle it.

In each of these cases the persons who felt attacked by weightist messages journeyed inside themselves and used the cycles to regain their inner balance. Yes, it hurts to be ridiculed. Yes, it is sad and infuriating that people make assumptions about one's value and control on the basis of weight. But those are their problems, not yours. You have no control over their weightism. Your challenge is to take away their power to hurt you by avoiding your own weightist thoughts.

The Body Pride Cycle, Part 2

Using words, not my weight, to express myself

I learned about emotional overeating early in my life, not only from my own adolescent cravings for cinnamon rolls and pumpkin pie, but later from books and piles of journal articles on the subject.

It seemed that on both a personal and a professional level, I understood something about the role of emotional overeating as a driving force behind weight gain. What took me far longer to appreciate was the perhaps equally important role of *the drive to stay heavy*. Body size speaks in paragraphs. As such, maintaining a particular size can have a hidden advantage.

It was Jack Obedzinski, a behavioral pediatrics professor at the university, who introduced me to this powerful dynamic when he presented at a seminar the fascinating case of a young boy . . .

There was a hidden advantage for this boy . . .

James, a 12-year-old, had suffered a serious hip injury playing soccer and to recover was forced to stay on the couch or in a wheelchair. This boy was from a loving family, but there were five children, and as the passive middle child, James, was the last to receive his parents' attention and affection.

Things changed when James was injured. Both his mother and his father flooded him with attention. His father brought him candy. His mother rented any video he wanted. And three months after his original injury, James was still not back at school, and still needed a wheelchair.

Jack explained that although James desperately wanted to see his friends at school, play ball and ride his bike, nothing he did seemed to heal his hip. With Jack's help, his parents realized that being in a wheelchair served an unconscious purpose for James. Hip pain and the inability to walk were how James told his family, "I need attention."

What was so riveting was the impact of James using words to express himself instead of using his pain and the wheelchair to do it for him. Once he could say, in words, "I need attention," his parents could make amends. They told him they realized he hadn't received the attention he deserved and said they wanted him to get well.

Two weeks later, James's pain was gone and he returned to school. He didn't need to be in a wheelchair any longer in order to express himself.

The hidden benefits of body size

The same dynamic is at work in the situation of weight. We want to lose weight, but there is a silent voice in us that speaks louder than we do, operating as the Wizard of Oz did, behind the green curtain.

Maintaining a body size larger than our biologic comfort zone is how we send wordless messages to others. Even if we spend years dieting and sweating off pounds, this voice will express itself through a relentless sabotage that results in weight staying rock solid.

Little or none of this is conscious. We don't *purposely* sabotage our healthy eating and scuttle our exercise plans to keep our weight high, *but it may still be happening*. We seem to spontaneously regain the weight without really knowing why.

What is our challenge? To give that voice words and sound so that it can speak directly and stop expressing itself through extra weight. For this reason, the second part of the body pride cycle is learning to use words instead of weight to express ourselves.

"I don't want you to know me. Stay away."

A robust woman with red hair, Charlotte was the secretary at the grammar school in my community. She was the most effusively sweet and caring woman you'd ever want to meet. Everyone loved her. So why with all that caring and appreciation from children and parents did she struggle and yet never seem to lose her extra weight?

In Charlotte's case, most of her weight issue had to do with genetics and periodic bouts of emotional overeating, yet the hidden advantage of staying larger than her body's biologic comfort zone definitely added to the persistence of her weight problem. For Charlotte, her body size said, "I don't want you to know me too well. If you did, you wouldn't like me, so give me some emotional distance."

In reality, everybody would have liked Charlotte just as much if she weren't quite as nice, but Charlotte pushed herself to be perfect, so she always felt somehow . . . fake. Her weight was a way of keeping people at bay so they wouldn't discover her flaws.

Charlotte would never have shared this kind of sensitive information with a group, but in our private sessions together she told me, "I don't want to be close to people. I don't want anyone to know me that well. What my weight says for me is: 'Don't know me. Keep a certain distance from me.'"

Just hearing herself say that shocked Charlotte because she had always considered herself such a warm and open person. She realized that she wasn't very warm to herself, and that began a chain of events that led her to approach herself in a more accepting way. At that point, Charlotte didn't need those extra pounds anymore, and right then her eating plans and exercise program seemed to start working.

"I feel powerless. Taking up space gives me power."

Jack, a lawyer with three partners from his grammar school days, volunteered that his weight was a way of showing power. It wasn't that he didn't have power, because he did. But despite his external successes—money, recognition and status—there was still a part of him that often had difficulty assuming the adult role and still felt unimportant and weak.

Jack told me he had a hint that there might be an advantage to his staying heavy. Each time he lost weight, he felt very vulnerable. Quickly he regained every ounce of it. Moreover, he was conscious that he liked being big. Taking up space in a room made him feel *stronger*.

What Jack needed was to use words, not his weight, to express himself. When he began saying to himself, "I feel powerless and I need my weight to feel more powerful," he scoffed at himself. "I should feel powerful because of my work and money situation, but the fact is, I don't." He shook his head. "Being big is not the most effective way to express my need to feel power. It just makes me less healthy and less agile."

With this revelation, Jack appeared to relax. He began reflecting on the facade he had put up and coming to terms with a childhood in which he had felt alone and powerless. After using words, not weight, to express himself, Jack could reexamine his sense of powerlessness for its own sake because it was out in the open and not wrapped up with the issue of weight.

When I happened to see Jack at a social event eight months later, he looked markedly leaner. He pulled me aside and eagerly updated me on his progress. According to Jack, it had taken him several months to find a new internal equilibrium that allowed him to feel powerful without his extra body fat. He said that when that leap occurred for him, it was as if his appetite "turned off." He didn't want to overeat anymore because his weight had outlived its purpose.

"Don't expect too much from me."

Nina was pretty, a brown-haired woman who taught preschool and spoke in a quiet voice. Her clothes, her hair and her posture all said the same thing: don't notice me, don't expect much from me, I don't want to disappoint you. So did her weight.

What surprised me about Nina was that when she realized she was using her weight to announce to the world that she was average and no more, she was aghast.

What does your weight say for you?

Don't notice me.
I am not important.
I am powerful.
I feel powerless.
I am a good mother.
Feel sorry for me.
I don't want sex.
I am stable and dependable.
Don't mess with me.
Don't expect too much of me.
I am not perfect.
Stay away from me.
I feel angry.
I am afraid to be all I can be.
I am not worthy.
I have given up.
I am loyal to my family.
I don't want to grow up.
I don't want you to judge me.
I reject you.
I need space.
I need love.

She knew she was a great teacher and an excellent mother and an incredibly loving wife. Why would she be trying to give off the message that she didn't have much to offer?

She was right. None of this was *logical*, but the part of us stuck below the separation of the generations line isn't logical, and that part of Nina took a certain comfort in pitying herself and reveling in her sense of inadequacy. It was a familiar feeling to her because that's how she'd felt growing up. The reality was that Nina had become an exceptional person—but her self-image had not caught up with the current truth.

When Nina saw how foolish she was in viewing herself as the frightened, inadequate child she had been rather than the extremely competent woman she had become, she began to readjust her thinking. Why shouldn't people notice her? Why shouldn't they expect good things from her?

Nina's appearance then changed. She highlighted her hair, switched to colorful clothing, put on some tasteful jewelry and starting having fun with her appearance. She didn't want to be invisible anymore, and she wanted people to expect something of her. That's when she began to lose weight.

"I don't want to make love."

Carol, a wildly successful entrepreneur, was unhappy in her marriage. Ben was a good husband and she had no thoughts of leaving him, but more and more they were emotionally estranged. The conflict arose because as Carol received less on an emotional level from Ben, she desired him less.

As is often the case, the less Carol wanted to make love, the more Ben wanted to and the more disappointed he became when they found time for it so infrequently. Carol didn't want to hurt Ben by rejecting him directly but couldn't help but notice that as her weight increased, Ben's insistence on frequent passionate encounters subsided. Before long, weight became an advantage to Carol because it said without words, "I don't want sex."

For Carol to quiet this drive to maintain her higher weight, she had to use those words to express herself. What she did was to go to Ben and say, "I care for you, but we've grown apart, so I don't desire you as much. I want to regain that closeness with you, and I don't want to make love with you until I do."

There, it was said. How relieved Carol was because now she could settle into improving the emotional foundation of her marriage without keeping her weight artificially high to protect her from unwanted advances. She could take off that weight without feeling so vulnerable.

"I'm so mad at you that I'll stay heavy."

Bruce gained weight initially because of his promotion at work and the difficulty he had setting limits with restaurant food. But when his wife, Nancy, began obvious manipulations to make him lose weight, he was deeply insulted.

Thus began a power struggle. Nancy fixed diet foods at home and swept the kitchen cupboards clean of all his favorite foods. Bruce found a reason to plan business lunches at which saying no to delectable foods would be hard for even the most committed health enthusiast. Keeping on those twenty pounds became a way for Bruce to say, "Nancy, you can't control me."

Bruce's pattern is a common one. Often people keep on weight as a sign of rebellion, just to show a father, wife or friend that they won't alter their body just to please them. Ironically, they're still giving control of their body size to another person; it's just that they're pumping up the size of their body rather than whittling it down. When people discover that in an effort to gain control, they've actually given their control away, they're usually dumbfounded.

When Bruce recognized that he was using staying overweight to show his anger at Nancy, he laughed. "I really outsmarted her, didn't I?" were his precise words, and what followed was an intense conversation between Bruce and Nancy during which he dealt with the real issue. He told Nancy, "I don't want you to control me. I need you to focus on yourself and not on trying to fix or perfect me." Soon after Bruce used words rather than weight to express himself, his weight plummeted.

A little warmth and curiosity makes all the difference.

Obviously, our weight speaks to the world in paragraphs, not just sentences. If you maintain a slight distance from this part of the cycle, saying to yourself, "*I wonder what my weight says for me now?*" you'll probably come back to this question over and over again, and come up with a different answer each time.

All the sentiments that your weight communicates for you can be brought to your awareness and expressed verbally. Each time you use words, not your weight, to express yourself, you'll *need* the extra weight less. Then it becomes easier and easier to attain the weight you've determined is best for your health and happiness.

The Body Pride Cycle, Part 3

Honoring and accepting my body

At the beginning of this chapter, we talked about how body and soul, mind and matter are intertwined, making the ultimate goal of the body pride cure acceptance of both body and self. How many people do you know, even those in midlife and beyond, who actually accept themselves? Admittedly, this is a huge developmental leap, but it can be broken down into small steps, which you take as you use the method and the tools I show you in this chapter.

Let's begin with acceptance.

Most of us have no difficulty accepting our good or light side—being able to sing on key, a knack for telling jokes, a sharp memory or a warmth that relaxes others. What about the rest? The flaws, imperfections, and inadequacies that we ignore, despise or incessantly try to change to no avail. That dark side is the target of this part of the body pride cycle.

We begin by questioning whether we *should* accept this dark side.

A good question. Hating those qualities doesn't make them disappear, but why accept them? It sounds as if we're planning our own mediocrity. Hardly. We're giving ourselves the opportunity to get off the fence, to change something we don't like about ourselves rather than living in a chronic state of low-level self-rejection.

Just five things . . .

In the training for the Solution groups, we use a very effective tool: Just Five Things. It asks you to identify things you *do* and *don't* like about your body and self. This tool prompts you to come to a decision: Among those qualities you don't like, are any changeable? If yes, will you change or accept them? If they are not changeable, grieve the loss involved, and accept that part of yourself.

Stacy's acceptance of her body and herself

When Stacy and I worked through her Just Five Things, she immediately jumped in with a list of what she didn't like about her body: her frizzy hair, scarred knee, round stomach, husky thighs and many freckles. Nor was she fond of her bouts of depression, looseness with money, laziness when it came to housework, bad attitude toward exercise and difficulty with procrastination.

On the positive side, she liked her large eyes, strong fingernails, graceful neck, straight teeth and round breasts. Moreover, she had a number of personal qualities she liked, which centered around her humor, kindness and generosity.

Stacy's first challenge was to take seriously the negative characteristics she had decided to change—instead of living with them, to change them. Her second challenge was to face those areas she didn't accept but couldn't change, in order to avoid further self-rejection. Her task was to focus directly on those qualities, grieve the losses they represented and let them go, letting the peacefulness of acceptance flood into her being.

Of course, this is not at all easy to do.

It was her stomach that she continued to reject.

As Stacy worked through the process of sorting out what she would change and what she would accept, she hit a rough patch. She knew that even if she lost almost all her extra weight, she had gained so much in the past that her stomach would never look the way it did when she was younger. She said in our group: "There's nothing I can do about my stretch marks. My body is lumpy and full because that's how all the women in our family are. I could have liposuction, but I can't afford it and I really don't want that. What I want is to accept my hips and see them as a part of me. I've lost some weight, so they are definitely smaller and I can wear pants and look pretty good,

Just Five Things

I like about *myself*:	I don't like about *myself*:
1.	1.
2.	2.
3.	3.
4.	4.
5.	5.

I like about my *body*:	I don't like about my *body*:
1.	1.
2.	2.
3.	3.
4.	4.
5.	5.

- Pause and appreciate the things you like.
- Of the things you don't like:
  Which are possible to change?
  Of those that are *possible* to change, which will you change?
  Of those that are *not possible* to change, which will you accept?

so I want to get over the hip rejection. I don't think I'll ever be in love with my hips, but think I can honor them."

Compassion and acceptance are contagious . . .

This led to a positive contagion in the group, with others musing over the previously hated parts of their bodies and selves. Nearly everyone in the group drew on this compassionate spirit and found things they were ready to accept about themselves.

For some, that involved some grieving. Stacy, in particular, had flare-ups of dissatisfaction with her hips, and she grieved the loss by writing Feelings Letters. They brought her through the range of emotions to acceptance and worked very well for her. According to Stacy: "Coming to peace with my body is a slow process. But it's already changing the quality of my life. I used to cover up with jackets and loose clothes. I think of that now and wince because I treated my body as if it was shameful. I know that if I hadn't accepted my hips, in particular, I would have passed all that dieting anxiety and body rejection onto my daughter. How sad that would have been."

There was another notion: honoring the body.

After Stacy came more to terms with her body and herself, savoring the parts she liked and either changing or accepting the ones she didn't like, a question of honor remained. For the last part of the body pride cycle involves not just accepting the body and self, but honoring them, esteeming them, valuing them.

It's ultimately necessary that we honor, esteem and value ourselves so that we'll engage in all the necessary, but largely invisible, acts required to take care of our health and our happiness. When we honor, esteem and value ourselves, we behave more like the hardware store clerk with a stake in the store's profits who chases after the customer who left his sunglasses on the counter. We act less like the summer help who shoves those sunglasses into a drawer.

We will go that extra—and completely necessary—mile to take care of ourselves.

Finding that sense of honoring of the body and self has many possible origins, but two are most common. One is based in the mind; the other in the soul.

Stanley was logical about it.

Honoring the self begins with the idea that nobody cares more about you than you. If you don't honor yourself, *who will*? That was the approach taken by Stanley, the family doctor at San Francisco General Hospital:

"I've worked enough in hospitals to know that nobody cares more about whether the doctor amputates the correct leg than the patient who is under the knife. It's not that I don't trust people, it's just that I'm realistic. Each person's number one job is to take care of themselves.

"If I do a sloppy job of minding what I eat or whether I've had enough exercise that day, there's no one out there who's going to tap me on the shoulder and say, 'You're not taking care of yourself.' It's my role to honor myself because I'm the person who cares the most about me."

To Donna, body pride was a spiritual matter.

For Donna, who raises Arabian horses and was an adored child growing up, honoring her body was a spiritual matter. She viewed her body as the worldly expression of her soul. As a result, she saw caring for and taking pride in her body as a way of showing spiritual devotion.

"I'm not an objectively beautiful woman, but my life is precious and if I've been given life, I want to value it. If I abuse my body or neglect my appearance, I'm not honoring the gift of life or the spirit I have inside me. The reality is that I enjoy honoring my body as a way of showing I appreciate life and am aware of my spiritual nature."

Whatever your reason for honoring your body and yourself, it's time to consider making a personal decision that—despite the flaws and imperfections—you are not only perfectly acceptable, but more than enough, right now, in this time and place. The experience of life is solitary no matter how much intimacy we achieve with others. There will never be another you.

Consider the possibility of honoring yourself *for no logical reason* other than that you exist, you feel and you are. And that your body will not always be. You require tending and acceptance and respect to thrive, and there is no one on earth who can give that to you but you.

> **Are you willing to honor and accept your body and yourself?**

Arriving from the opposite direction: external changes

There is another route to enhancing our body pride. We can *fake it until we make it.* In other words, it is possible for us to move and dress with pride without having yet achieved a full-blown sense of body pride. By standing, moving and dressing with body pride we enhance our positive view of ourselves.

If you were to put on your favorite outfit, groom until you're gorgeous all over and stand as if you were Princess Di, Whitney Houston and Sylvester Stallone all wrapped into one, what would happen to your body pride? It would become stronger!

Isn't this just lookism? How superficial! It's not the body that counts, but the mind, heart and soul. Who cares if you're body proud? *You do.* Because of the inevitable intermingling of self and body, the way you regard and treat your body *matters.*

I can remember buying three pants suits in the early seventies for a job I had landed in San Francisco's financial district. Although they had a price tag far above my budget, the suits were drab and masculine, which was just right for me and for many women negotiating a place in the mainly male work environment. I

Experiment! What is the effect on your body pride of . . .

slouching over	vs.	standing tall?
a shuffling step	vs.	a brisk step?
shabby clothes	vs.	glorious attire?

didn't want to dress to please men or deal with romantic advances, and I wanted to be taken *seriously*.

Then one day I met a woman who saw things differently. She was a pretty redhead, who took great joy in her looks. She wore tasteful accessories, impeccable makeup and elegant, eye-catching clothes. I didn't ask her about her attitude toward her appearance; she told me. "Laurel, why don't you enjoy your appearance more? You're not dressing to get a *reaction*. You're dressing for *yourself*, because it's fun to enjoy your appearance, to adorn yourself and to have fun being a woman. It's something you do to celebrate yourself."

Dress, groom and move with self-love and body pride.

Her approach was *completely* foreign to me, but I began to see that I had *given away* my power to others—completely unintentionally. I had chosen drab, concealing clothes, wore little makeup and adopted a certain slouch that conveyed the message "Don't notice me." The idea of seeing myself anew and shaping my appearance for *my own* enjoyment was nothing less than exciting.

If you're willing, begin a process of looking at yourself anew. In truth, you *are* new, just as we all are each day. What could you do in your grooming, dressing and moving to show that you honor yourself and take pride in your body? Here are the actions some of our group members took as they renewed their body pride:

"I cleaned out my whole closet and got rid of all the clothes that I wore in order to say, 'Don't look at me.'"

"On Mondays I dress as if my appearance really matters. It feels good and it's a great way to put me in a good mood for the week."

"I get a manicure every Friday, and I completely redid my makeup and jewelry to be more eye-catching. I'm treating myself as if I matter. I love it."

"I realized that my clothes made me look old before my time. I bought pleated pants and some cowboy boots too, just for the fun of it."

The tremendous effect of standing body proud.

A few years ago, I took a walk around Phoenix Lake, a little punch bowl of water nestled in Mount Tamalpais near my home, with David Surrenda, a mind-body health authority, on the suggestion of a mutual friend who said we *must* meet.

In the midst of a rather philosophical conversation, he commented on my walk. I had a "stovepipe" walk, according to him, with straight legs pounding on the earth. I didn't know whether to laugh at such a remark or to listen. What I did was laugh. Then I listened.

And as we finished our loop around the lake, David, who is a psychologist by training, explained to me the power of the way one stands and moves. Not only is it a message to the outer world, but more important, it's a message to yourself.

Pretending it doesn't matter how you stand or how you move suggests that *you* don't matter. And so I learned and I tried to improve my slumpy posture, using what I call the body pride stance, pictured on page 243, which was developed by Suki Munsell, Ph.D. In addition, I made an effort to notice my walk, moving a little more smoothly, and realized that how I moved mattered.

According to Gloria Steinem in *Revolution from Within,* "Women in particular need to understand how something as simple as physical posture can undermine, or enhance, self-confidence. In the unified body-mind field of the self, the movement of any molecule shifts the others."

To my surprise, when I applied these ideas to myself, it had a *remarkable* effect. When I stood and walked as if I mattered, as if I weren't invisible and as if I honored myself, I felt better. Each time I consciously stood with body pride, I was feeding my sense of my own worth. Consider using these tools yourself. Just jump in and experiment with them. Notice the effects they have on your attitude toward your body and self.

What changes will you make in standing, moving, grooming or dressing?

Gathering up your own body pride . . .

Just by reading this chapter, you're likely to begin ridding yourself of the inner villain of weightist thoughts and supplanting

The Body Pride Stance

Begin by . . .
Stand with feet parallel, walking distance apart. Roll down, first chin to chest, then allowing your hands to reach down toward the ground.

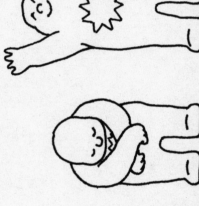

Then . . .
Cross your wrists as if you were grabbing onto a long shirt. Roll up, pulling the shirt off over your head.

Last . . .
Reach your arms overhead and stretch, elongating your entire body.

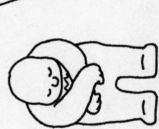

Body Pride!
Slowly lower your arms to your sides, still growing tall. Soften your knees. Tuck your pelvis under and stand tall with body pride!

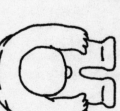

them with body pride statements. Perhaps you have become conscious of using words rather than weight to express yourself. And understand that the very heart of the matter of body pride is acceptance and honoring of both the body and the self.

Now your task is to be very patient and gentle with yourself as you slowly master this cure. It may help to keep in mind the image of a master craftsperson slowly refinishing the finest antique wood, taking it one layer at a time. Like your body pride, when the piece is finally finished it radiates a satiny luster that is created only through persistence and a great deal of patience.

Cure 4. Good Health

Of all the cures, the only one that I catch myself resisting is the good health cure. It seems not only a little boring, but somewhat maddening.

Whenever we talk about the good health cycle in a group meeting, the reaction among participants is almost always the same: heavy silence, mild annoyance and a modicum of guilt.

Cure 4. Good Health

Optimizing your physical vitality.

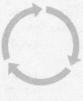

3. Health
Care

1. Body
Awareness

2. Self-Care

"If only I treated my body as well as I treat my car!"

Jennifer was largely unaware of her body and had little if any commitment to taking care of it. At 28 she had the glamorous job of production assistant for a film company, often working fourteen-hour days without breaking for more than coffee and candy bars. At night she blew off the stress of the day with wine, fast food and reruns of old movies.

Jennifer said to the group with a self-accepting laugh, "I don't bother with my health. If my car turns over a little rough in the morning, I don't mind being late to work. I take my car in immediately. Yet if my stomach hurts or my head aches, what do I do? Deny it! I completely ignore it until it's so bad that I have no choice whatsoever but to do something about it. I know that without my vitality, nothing is good, but I still don't treat my body as well as I treat my car!"

According to David Surrenda, Ph.D., a wellness consultant to major corporations of Silicon Valley, "People have a sense of whether they're healthy or not. They know if something's going wrong, but the background noise is so loud that they can't hear it."

In Jennifer's case, the background noise of her lifestyle and her emotional resistance to tending to her health kept her from noticing and taking care of small health problems as they arose.

"I don't want to deal with my health. I'm only 28 and I think I have a couple of decades before things will go too far wrong. I don't want to go to the doctor because I don't want any bad news. And those little symptoms? They usually go away or I take Tylenol and don't worry about them."

Jennifer's reasoning sounds normal and is perfectly understandable, given the common barriers that cause us to be lax about taking care of our health:

- I'm too busy.
- There are costs involved.
- I don't like my doctor.

- It's hard to get off work.

- Whatever advice I get won't be good.

- The questions are embarrassing and intrusive.

- It takes time to get an appointment.

- I don't like not being in control.

- I'm afraid of what I'll hear.

Often the reason the barriers seem insurmountable is the emotional intensity that underlies all health issues. After all, no one is getting out of this life alive, and we all decline and perish.

You and I can never solve our weight problem if we are not well. When the body is on the blink, so is the rest of life. Our emotional, physical and practical needs go unmet, and life takes a downturn, making going to the gym unlikely and eating for health a low priority.

> "I have chronic back pain and it makes me tired, so I go to bed early."

> "I feel fine except my body is so stiff. Then I get these tension headaches at work and it blows the whole day."

> "I don't take my blood pressure pills, but I worry about it all the time."

> "Estrogen replacement therapy made me gain weight, so I stopped it. Now I feel older and more lethargic."

The quickest route to health: taking out our emotional trash

All this sagging vitality is not the result of lapses in medical know-how. The lapse is within us, and we have good reason for it. Being sick is frightening. Getting help is not only tiresome, expensive and time-consuming, but in the end may not work. Do we really want to give control of our bodies to someone else, whom we don't always trust? Are we capable of finding our own answers, and if we had them would we act on them?

In order to truly take care of our health, we need to find and express the complex feelings that arise when we suspect that our health is in danger. We must deal not only with our current emotional reaction to illness but with the angers, hurts, fears and guilts we carry from our past experiences with medical care. The release of these feelings is the straightest route to taking care of our health and attaining maximum vitality.

Jennifer returned herself to balance.

Jennifer used the nurturing and limits cycles. Like all of us, when she wasn't taking care of her health she was stuck in the child role, acting out the rebellious, irresponsible side we all have inside us to some extent.

Watch how using these cycles brought Jennifer back into her adult role, so she was motivated to take care of her personal vitality.

The Nurturing Cycle

I feel . . . tired a lot. I feel lethargic and I get headaches at work. I worry that I'm anemic or maybe I have multiple sclerosis or cancer. I feel angry that my body isn't stronger and healthier. Other people live the way I do and they feel fine.

I need . . . to get more sleep. To go to bed by midnight. To get more exercise. To get a checkup, but I don't have a doctor I like. I need a new doctor.

Would you please . . . (say to the clerk at the medical clinic) I would like to try a new doctor here. I would prefer a woman. Can you suggest one and give me an appointment?

The Limits Cycle

I expect . . . to find out that there is something really wrong with me. Is that a reasonable expectation? No. I'm still young and I don't have any unusual symptoms. A reasonable expectation would be that I may have something small wrong with me.

I think . . . that going to the doctor is a waste of time. Are those thoughts helping? No. What could I say to myself that would be positive and powerful, so I would follow through and go the the appointment? I need to take care of my health. Getting some feedback and information is important. It won't take that much time.

The essential pain . . . is that I could get some bad news or have an appointment that isn't helpful. What feeling arises from that? Fear and anger. I need to sit with those feelings for a while. Fear and anger. They are beginning to fade. Will I follow through with going to my appointment? Yes, I think so.

Jennifer *did* go to the appointment and she *did* find out that she was anemic, and she was also given some relaxation techniques to cut down on her headaches. Her new physician changed her contraceptive pills because of side effects, and she discovered that her blood pressure was, in fact, very good. To the group she announced that she was really proud that she had gone.

The good health cycle involves first being aware of your body, then doing what you can to optimize your health, and last, making sure that your health care is effective.

The Good Health Cure, Part 1
How does my body feel?

The first part of the cure is to be aware of your physical health every day. This awareness in not a quick check to determine if there is pain, blood or fever, but a more sensitive scan of your body that will pick up subtle signs of body difficulties before they become serious.

Scan your body from head to toe right now.

What good feelings do you notice? What uncomfortable feelings do you sense?

The body scan technique helps you mentally review each part of your body from head to toe, appreciating your body's good feelings and listening to your body's feelings. It sounds simple, but Jennifer didn't find scanning her body easy.

"Why would I spend my time noticing my body?"

"My work is very hectic. I feel like I'm running up against deadlines constantly, so most of the time I'm thinking about what I'm trying to accomplish, and the furthest thing from my mind is my health. The idea of disconnecting from my thoughts and scanning my body seems odd. Why would I spend my time noticing the feelings in my body?"

We practiced the technique in the group, and with the social pressure of anticipating that everyone in the group would use the body scan that week, Jennifer tried it. The next week she told the group:

"When I began using the body scan technique, I noticed some good feelings I wasn't even aware of, like wiggling my toes and how relaxed my arms and legs are. I also saw where I carry my tension—in my neck and shoulders. No wonder I get so many headaches. When I realized that, I began stretching and moving my shoulders and neck during the day, and I didn't have those headaches the rest of the week! It is hard for me to mentally disconnect from the work pressures and scan my body, but I really need to do it more often."

The Body Scan

Every day, mentally scan your body from the top of your head to the tips of your toes.

Appreciate your body's <u>good</u> feelings.

*"Where do I feel
relaxed, strong, comfortable, sensuous,
healthy or good?"*

Listen to your body's <u>difficult</u> feelings.

*"Where do I feel
tense, weak, uncomfortable, numb,
unhealthy or bad?"*

Checking your body daily is an ingredient essential to your health, whether you do it at a specific time each day, such as when drying off after a shower, waking up in the morning or going to sleep at night, or periodically turn down the background noise of life long enough to become aware of the small sources of comfort and discomfort in your body. So much pain is avoided and so much vitality is gained if we do this simple thing. Here are a few experiences from the lives of patients in the program:

> "I didn't listen to that pain in my back. I just kept increasing the weights in my workout. Now I pulled this muscle and I can't exercise for two months."

> "I get back pain every time my mother visits. It's stress, I know it is. If I don't catch the first signs of the pain and do some yoga or stretching or just take time away from my mother, the pain takes hold and I have it for a week after she leaves."

> "I noticed I felt sleepy and I didn't do anything about it. I was chronically underrested like the rest of the human race. Then I had three small accidents in a row: one in my car and two mishaps in which I bumped into something at work. The auto accident cost me $500. I should have listened to my body."

When will you scan your body each day?

The Good Health Cure, Part 2

Am I taking care of my body?

Much of what is required to take care of your health is already part of the method. Eating well and living an active, fulfilling life go a long way toward preventing and treating health problems. But there is more you must do. Scanning the body reveals information that prompts us to take action. A blister on the heel needs a bandage, and tension in the neck requires a gentle massage.

When you become aware that you aren't well, you must take action to ensure the return of vitality. Some things you can do yourself. Others require help from your health care providers.

Am I in denial or a hypochondriac?

The problem is that it's sometimes hard to know how we feel physically, even when we do take time to scan our bodies. If we've been raised in a permissive or depriving way, we may be unaware not just of our emotions, but of our physical self as well. As a result, we might deny or minimize problems—or exaggerate them. After years of ignoring or misreading our bodies, we find our intrinsic wisdom has been blocked.

- "Every time I get a headache, somewhere deep inside me I know it's brain cancer."

- "I thought, Me? It's just a stomachache. Or maybe it's a little indigestion. It turned out to be an ulcer."

And if those who raised us weren't skilled at honoring our boundaries and control, we may find the intimate arena of medical services somewhat frightening.

- "I can take care of my own health. I don't let a doctor near me. They do more harm than good."

- "If I go to a doctor, they'll make me do things I don't want to do. I solve the problem by not going at all."

The buck stops with you.

Regardless of issues of control, self-awareness or emotions, the responsibility to keep yourself full of vitality and as free as possible from disease rests with you.

Typically a combination of self-care, alternative therapies and conventional treatments gives the best results. Your job, therefore, is to become your doctor's boss.

Doctors spend much of their time prescribing pills, so if you think other combinations of therapies may be cheaper, less risky and possibly more effective, you need to do your own homework about the health problems that crop up in your life—whether they're back troubles, PMS, recurrent infections or skin rashes.

Headaches were a factor in the weight of Lisa, a young Hispanic woman who couldn't go to work because of migraines.

Eating was the only thing that settled Lisa's stomach

during her three-day bouts of blinding pain, so she initially took no medicine for them. Eventually she began taking migraine pills, which helped her, but it was only when she combined the medication with several other therapies, including relaxation and yoga, that she saw real improvement. She read books, talked to friends, surfed the Internet and experimented with various techniques—efforts that led to an optimal blend of self-care and conventional medical care.

The basics of good health

The charts in this chapter provide some very basic information about taking care of your health and using medical care to your advantage as you solve your weight problem:

- *Basic self-care*—the tests and care you need to maintain health

- *Problems that promote weight gain*—a list of common medical conditions and how they affect weight

- *Drugs that promote weight gain*—drugs that add weight and how they do it

- *Drugs that promote weight loss*—their risks and mechanisms

This information is meant to give you a starting place, so that when you approach your physician you'll be better prepared to ask questions and get answers.

Self-care

The chart on pages 254–255 lists some of the tests, evaluations and treatments currently considered basic screening for health. If you haven't yet taken the tests and treatments indicated, please make an appointment with your doctor to do so right away.

Health problems and drugs may add to your weight.

It's not enough just to screen for health problems. You may already have health problems that make weight loss more difficult

Basic Self-Care

Check your:

Blood pressure	Every year and more often if it is high.
Cholesterol test	Every five years and more often if it is high.
Immunizations	A tetanus-diptheria shot every ten years; if 65 or older, a pneumonia shot once and a flu shot every year.
Teeth and gums	Regular dental checkups, brush after meals, floss daily.
Rectal exam	If you are 50 years of age or older (stool blood and sigmoidoscopy tests).
Mouth exam	If now or in the past you have consumed a lot of alcohol or have smoked or chewed tobacco.
Skin exam	If you have had skin cancer in your family or a lot of sun exposure. Wear sunscreen.
AIDS (HIV)	If you had a blood transfusion between 1978 and 1985, have injected illegal drugs, have had multiple sexual partners or any male homosexual activity.
STD tests	If you have had multiple sexual partners or any sexually transmitted diseases.
Glucose test	If you carry your weight in the middle or high on your body,

have a family member with diabetes or have had diabetes during pregnancy.

Eye exam | Every two years. Yearly if you are over 60, over 40 and black, or have diabetes.

For Women

Breast exam | Yearly exam by a doctor and monthly self-exams.

Mammogram | Regularly by age 50 or before if your mother or sister had breast cancer.

Pap smear | Yearly Pap smears, and more often if you have had genital warts, sexually transmitted diseases, multiple sexual partners or abnormal Pap smears.

Estrogen | Discuss with your doctor at age 40 or before.

For Men

Prostate exam | If you are age 50 or older.

Testicular exam | If you are age 15 to 35, particularly if you have had an atrophic or undescended testicle.

Aspirin therapy | If you are 40 years of age or older, discuss with your doctor.

Adapted from Dickey, LL, DiGuiseppe, C, and Atkins, D. Preventive Medicine I. Monograph, Edition No. 199, *Home Self-Assessment Program.* Kansas City, Mo.: American Academy of Family Physicians, December 1995.

(see page 257). If you do, it's important that you return to your physician to explore the range of ways these health problems can be effectively treated.

If your physician is apathetic ("It comes with age," "It's better than it was," or "It's not so bad"), find another doctor whose goal is not just to keep you alive but to support you in achieving maximum vitality!

Medications that heal us may also add to our body size. Sometimes a specific medication is our only health option, but often other medications can make us feel better without increasing our body weight. On page 258 is a list of medications that increase weight in some people. If you are taking one or more of them, please talk with your physician and pharmacist about substituting other options.

Should you take drugs for weight loss?

This is a personal decision. Weight-loss drugs work only for some people and only while they are taking them. Such drugs can never stimulate a weight solution, because they do not quiet all the mind and body drives to gain weight.

Information about weight-loss drugs approved by the Food and Drug Administration appears on page 259. Note their side effects and risks. Other drugs are sold without FDA approval because they are considered nutritional supplements or herbal preparations, not drugs. Many, therefore, have not been formally evaluated. Their purity and effeciveness are less well documented, and there is no guarantee of their safety. The FDA has withdrawn approval from many of these products—and taken them off the market—in the last ten years because of concerns about their safety or effectiveness. Before using any of these products, consult a physician, pharmacist or registered dietitian.

Consider both the immediate and long-term side effects of these drugs.

Even if you are considering use of FDA-approved weight-loss medications on only a short-term basis, examine the risks involved. As you can see, many side effects can occur, and this may be only a partial list. In addition, since most are relatively new drugs, not all the long-term effects are known. This is of par-

Problems That May Promote *Weight Gain*

The problems:	How they can affect weight
bone or joint troubles	you exercise less.
muscle injuries	you exercise less.
headaches	you exercise less.
chronic pain	you eat more or exercise less.
asthma	you exercise less because it is uncomfortable or unsafe.
allergies	you exercise less because you don't go outdoors.
chest pain	you exercise less because of concern that it isn't safe.
thyroid problems	you burn fewer calories.
PMS*	you eat more because you crave carbohydrates (affects 60 percent of women).
SAD**	you overeat and are less active (affects 30 percent of people).
tobacco withdrawal	you eat more due to carbohydrate cravings.
alcohol withdrawal	you eat more due to carbohydrate cravings.
substance abuse	you eat more due to carbohydrate cravings.
PTSS***	you eat more due to carbohydrate cravings.
depression	you eat more and exercise less.

* premenstrual syndrome, ** seasonal affective disorder, or "winter blues," *** post-traumatic stress syndrome

Drugs That May Promote *Weight Gain*

How they work	Type of drug	Examples
water retention	alpha adrenergic blocking agents	prazosin, terazosin
	steroid anti-inflammatories	prednisone
	NSAIDS*	naproxen, ibuprofen
	antidiabetic agents	chlorpropamide
	antithyroid	propylthiouracil
	antimania	lithium
	vasodilators	minoxidil
	antipsychotic	perphenazine
	female sex hormones	estrogen, progesterone
increased appetite	steroid anti-inflammatories	prednisone
	antidiabetic agents	insulin, glyburide
	antimania	lithium
	antidepressant	imipramine, sertraline
	antipsychotic	chlorpromazine
	female sex hormones	estrogen, progesterone
decreased activity	sedatives	flurazepam, temazepam
	tranquilizers	diazepam, chlordiazepoxide
		phenobarbital
	antihistamines	chlorpheniramine
		diphenhydramine

* nonsteroidal anti-inflammatories

Drugs That May Promote Weight Loss

How they work	Risks	Examples
Increase the availability to the brain of serotonin, a substance that decreases food intake. It has a calming (downer) effect.	Dry mouth, constipation, headache, sleep disturbance, memory and thinking problems, libido changes, depression, blurred vision, diarrhea and primary pulmonary hypertension.	dexfenfluramine fenfluramine
Increase the availability of dopamine in places of the brain that cause a decrease in food intake. They have a stimulating (upper) effect.	Dry mouth, constipation, blurred vision, overstimulation, restlessness, sleep disturbance, headache, libido changes, tremor, increased blood pressure and tachycardia.	phentermine diethylpropion benzphetamine
Central nervous system stimulants (uppers) that boost metabolic rate.	Same as above except no libido changes.	caffeine* ephedrine* phenylpropanolamine*
Increase protein breakdown and oxygen use.	Loss of lean tissue, osteoporosis, and heart problems.	thyroid hormone
Loss of water from the body.	Loss of potassium, muscle cramps, and nausea.	caffeine* hydrochlorothiazide ammonium chloride

* nonprescription drug

ticular concern because these drugs are designed to affect the brain. Serious long-term side effects may include stimulating brain changes that make us more susceptible to depression and weight gain.

For instance, dexfenfluramine can cause primary pulmonary hypertension, a rare but sometimes fatal disorder, as well as a host of less serious side effects. Also, when animals were given ten times the human dosage of dexfenfluramine, their natural ability to produce serotonin was crippled. In humans, a drop in serotonin levels is associated with carbohydrate cravings. Moreover, the drug has undergone human testing for less than a year.

Last, the impact of these drugs on weight is not impressive. For instance, according to a study published in *The Lancet*, after a year of administering dexfenfluramine, weight had decreased only 3 percent of initial weight more than the weight of those taking a placebo or sugar pill, in this case about seven pounds. The weight loss with these drugs occurs in the first six months and requires that you continue to take the medication in order to maintain that rather small weight loss.

Moreover, although consumer interest in pills has been phenomenal—over 380,000 prescriptions were written for weight-loss drugs between April and September of 1996—about 75 percent of patients stop taking the pills.

Philosophical issues often arise.

Finally, we may have philosophical judgments or strong feelings about the wisdom of taking drugs. We should question these views and honor our conclusions.

One view is: Weight loss is hard. Why not make it easier to lose weight by taking drugs, and put our efforts toward more meaningful pursuits? Worry about your job, your kids or the environment, not your weight.

On the other hand, as Alain Ehrenbert, a sociologist, said in reference to mood-altering medications, which can be seen as analogous to weight-loss drugs: "The risk is creating a world without suffering that will make it harder for people to handle ordinary frustrations without chemical help."

Another point of view is: "Those drugs don't solve weight problems, they just give me an edge. If I have to solve the problem anyway, I might as well get at it and not bother with the risks and side effects of taking drugs."

In the end, whether or not you augment your weight solution with drugs is a very personal matter. Talk with your doctor and pharmacist, your friends and family. Use the nurturing and limits cycles to arrive at an answer that is right for you.

The Good Health Cure, Part 3

Is my health care effective?

For many of us it is easier to wrestle a lion to the ground than to negotiate today's health care system. If you become sick, simply getting the care you need can be an exhausting and overwhelming proposition.

The third part of the good health cycle is becoming proactive in guaranteeing that your health care needs are met. Since this will require phone calls, letters and forms, it will also most likely require that you make diligent use of the other cycles. The nurturing cycle can guide you through the inherent frustrations involved, and you can draw upon the limits cycle to ensure that your expectations are reasonable and your follow-through effective.

Preparing for your visit

Your doctor may have a reassuring bedside manner and impeccable medical judgment but still be prevented from providing you with the most sensitive and effective health care. Considering the changes in the health care system, it is even more critical that we approach a medical visit conscientiously, arriving well prepared, speaking effectively and following up carefully.

For most of us, preparation includes making a list. Why? Because these visits are rushed and emotionally charged. Often we leave the session and realize that we haven't discussed half our symptoms and issues.

The body scans that are part of this cycle give you ideal information with which to begin. Make a list of any unusual sensations or discomforts as well as any worries or concerns you have. List all over-the-counter and prescription medications you take.

Preparing to Visit Your Physician

1. **How do you feel?**
   Anger, sadness, fear and guilt are common.
   Feel and express those feelings.
2. **Check your body.**
   What feels good? What doesn't feel good?
3. **Make a list of questions.**
   What information, advice and referrals do you
   need?
4. **Bring the list with you to the visit.**
   Put it in your pocket or purse and take it to
   the visit

Add to the list your drug allergies. Consider any referrals you might need to further enhance your health.

Giving your physician a hamburger sandwich

We've dealt with the emotional barriers to getting our health care needs met. We've equipped ourselves with a list of the information, advice and referrals we want, and most important, we've remembered to bring the list to the session.

But when the doctor walks into the examining room we may shrivel into a small child or build a self-protective angry wall. We forget that our doctors are human and need our full cooperation to do their job. As we would with any vulnerable human, we need to make requests that are effective. In other words, should the visit become unsatisfactory, we need to give our doctor a "hamburger sandwich."

How do we speak to physicians so they can hear us? We approach them with respect but not subservience, first giving them some *sincere* white bread. For example, "I know you're stuck for time" gives an immediate message that we are approaching them with compassion and understanding of their

Making Requests of Physicians

Make an effective request of your doctor by giving him or her a hamburger sandwich, that is, an empathetic statement, your message, then another empathetic statement.

The white bread
I understand that you are busy.
I know you have patients waiting.

The meat
I feel confused.
I need you to say that again.
Would you please explain it using words I understand?

I feel worried about my weight.
I need your understanding and help.
Would you please tell me what weight services are covered?

I feel angry when you talk to me that way.
I need to be treated with respect.
Would you please refer me to another doctor?

The white bread
I appreciate your help.
I understand you are doing the best you can.

situation. Next we bring out the meat: our list of questions for information, advice and referrals. Drawing on phrases such as "*I feel* . . . ," "*I need* . . ." *and* "*Would you please* . . ." protects us from acting passive or aggressive and plants us firmly in assertion. We then close with another statement of appreciation and compassion.

Darcy didn't bother to use any of the request techniques because she was seen in the emergency room after midnight, given potent painkillers and told to go home and rest.

What Darcy really needed was a referral to get an MRI, an expensive test that her health care provider only rarely approved. Though clearly in pain and full of narcotics, she insisted on coming to the weekly group. We practiced assertion at each session, but still the provider kept putting Darcy off. Darcy, for her part, in her pain, confusion and fear about her condition, allowed them to put her off. By the time her provider approved the MRI, she had become so addicted to painkillers, it took nearly a month to wean herself off.

Finally Darcy used the art of effective requests.

When Darcy realized what had happened—that she had been in horrendous pain and was addicted to narcotic painrelievers—she was furious. It was only then that she used the art of making effective requests to her advantage.

When Darcy finally talked to her doctor, she said, "I understand you have your own rules, and I also know you care about patients and find it hard to see people getting poor treatment. I feel violated. By following these rules, I've suffered for three weeks and I've become hooked on these pills.

"I need several things: First I need the names of the regulating boards within both your organization and the state with whom I can file a complaint. Second, I need you to work with me to make weaning myself from these pills as painless as possible. Finally, I need a referral for psychological services so I can vent some of the distress this situation has caused me. I know you have done what you had to do and I appreciate that you are in a difficult situation."

According to Darcy, the physician was at first defensive, then sided with her and provided all the services she wanted. A month later, Darcy had rid her body of the pain medications, and the original pain had disappeared. The lesson she learned was to give people a hamburger sandwich *earlier* in the process of asking for the health care she needed.

After the visit, staying in balance

There is something intimate about a visit with the doctor. The preparation, the arousal of emotion and intellect, and the eventual climax and resolution of the visit can bear a distant resemblance to the act of making love. The analogy turns on the issues of trust and control, and the intensity, vulnerability and self-revelation that can arise in the physician/patient encounter.

Unfortunately, after the visit, as in more intimate encounters, we may . . . fall asleep . . . and not follow through with taking the actions indicated during the visit.

After the visit we are responsible not only for checking and expressing our feelings but for determining what we've learned and still need to learn. Moreover, it is our task to plan what actions we will take and to follow through.

My appreciation for the merits of this cure is renewed each time I hear those who have mastered the program, particularly those who approached this cure with little enthusiasm, tell me

---

After You Visit Your Physician

1. **How do you feel?**
   Anger, sadness, fear and guilt, relief and pride are common. Feel and express those feelings.

2. **What did you learn?**
   What do you know now that you didn't know before?

3. **What further information do you need?**
   What do you still need to know? How will you get that information?

4. **What actions do you need to take?**
   What do you need to do next? What are reasonable expectations for doing them?

how much enhancing their health has affected their weight and their happiness.

> "I don't have the backache anymore. I don't wake up with it. I don't have it at work, and I don't have it when I work out. It's so great to have no body pain."

> "Those pills I was taking were making me retain water. My doctor didn't even mention the side effect to me, but when I brought it up, she changed my prescription and I lost five pounds in a week."

> "I lived with allergies for years and took those pills that made me sleepy. I finally got some prescription pills, so I don't have either the allergy symptoms or the sleepiness. It's great."

Physical health that is optimal—for who you are at this time—isn't an afterthought but is absolutely central to your weight solution. To thrive, a nourished spirit must reside within a body that is well-fed with physical vitality.

Cure 5. Balanced Eating

If I picked up this book in order to solve my weight problem, I would probably turn immediately to the chapter on food. I'd say to myself, *"Are they—after all this talk about cures and solutions—going to stick me with a diet?"*

The answer is *no*. I will not tell you what to eat, nor do I advise you to let anyone else do so—just the way you wouldn't allow anyone to orchestrate your intimate life or tell you when to go to bed. Besides, chances are you already know *more than enough* about what you "should" eat to resolve your weight problem.

Cure 5: Balanced Eating

Eating for health and pleasure.

3. Health and Pleasure

1. Regular Meals

2. Hunger

What I will do is tell you the truth—which is that there are two eating skills that will be key players in your weight solution:

- Knowing when to eat for *pleasure*—that is, eat precisely what, when and as much as you want for no other reason than that you *really need* it. That's right. It's perfectly fine—and even desirable—to eat for pleasure alone.

- Knowing when to eat for *health*—that is, when you *don't really need* to eat for pleasure alone but to eat in a healthy way.

How do you know what to eat when:

Someone brings a chocolate cake to the office and it looks luscious?

There are two pieces of pizza left and they look very appealing?

You're wandering around the kitchen, thinking about getting something to eat?

I don't know the answers. But I do know how you can make your *own* decision—one that is right for you.

Surprisingly, the way to decide is easy because it's an inside job. *All you need to do is pause a moment.* In that moment you do yourself a tremendous favor. You move out of the child role—which the smell and taste and sight of fabulous food brings out in us all—and into a place above the separation of the generations line. In that adult role you can readily journey inside and decide what is right for you in that situation at that time. The answer will be very clear to you because you will be:

- *So sensitive to your needs from using the nurturing cycle*—that you will know if you need chips, cake or pasta. And so self-accepting that when you decide you really need to eat to excess, you will do so with joy.

- *So strong from using the limits cycle*—that when you don't really need to eat for pleasure alone, you will accept the essential pain of eating in a healthier way with little fanfare or discomfort. In fact, as you eat in a way that shows more respect for your body, you will probably feel the earned reward of pride.

It seems unnatural that we should *need* these skills. Babies notice hunger and snuggle to the breast, and it seems only right that you and I should have the same freedom and ease. Upon noticing we are hungry, we should have the license to go to the fridge, the cupboard or the market and choose whatever foods capture our imagination.

In our culture of diversity and abundance, life is not so easy. What is in the fridge, the cupboard or the market varies drastically in what it brings us in calories, fat, sugar and nutrients, as well as in satisfaction and pleasure. These are trade-offs only we can make because they involve our very basic and always changing feelings and needs. Only with an acute awareness of our feelings and needs can we balance our competing priorities of health and pleasure and be sensitive to our bodies' actual need for nutrition.

These decisions, such as *"Should I eat the last piece of pizza or skip it?"* are very important because, as I've mentioned, the difference between those gaining weight and those maintaining it is only about 50 calories a day—the equivalent of one large bite from that pizza slice. If you are generally vigilant in giving your body the food it needs from day to day, that bite of pizza or even the whole slice won't matter all. Yet if you habitually override your body's signals and overeat, your weight will increase. You may react by restricting your eating or indulging yourself with food, only to find that your body size remains larger than your genetics requires it to be.

In this chapter, I will first guide you through the important specifics of healthy nutrition without sheltering you from the reality that eating in a healthy way is not the cultural norm. To take good care of your personal nutrition may require you to have clear limits with others—that is, to choose a different nutritional pathway from that of your friends, relatives and co-workers.

I'm not suggesting that you eat foods that taste like bark off a tree, but that you be mindful of eating the healthy foods you enjoy. For example, who doesn't take pleasure from such healthy edibles as ripe strawberries, fresh bread, sweet corn, hot cereal, baked potatoes, crisp watermelon, chewy bagels or turkey sandwiches?

Then I will share with you a way to make decisions about when it is in your best interests to toss out your concern for the health benefits of your food and relish eating whatever delectable fare you desire at that moment—a hot fudge sundae, a cheeseburger or a slab of pie.

As you master the method, you will watch yourself begin to eat in a very natural, relaxed and pleasurable way even if you were taught to clean your plate or have measured your food for years. You will begin to trust that you can stop when you're satisfied and your body will compensate by giving out fewer hunger signals the next day.

We hear these comments over and over during our groups:

"I eat fast food for a night or two and something goes off inside me and I end up wanting a salad the third night."

"Candy is OK but I don't feel the same after eating it as I do after eating an apple. I stick to apples most of the time."

"I've had enough. I don't like the feeling of being too full."

Before you begin . . .

The balanced eating cure is easy and effective because it rests on the progress you have made with the other cures. With your moods more balanced and your body more active, your natural appetite regulation mechanisms take over and send you accurate signs of your need for food. If you obey these signs of hunger, eating when you are hungry and stopping when you are just satisfied, not full, your weight will decrease slowly and well.

However, in some situations your body's hunger signals may *not* be accurate. For instance, if you chronically overeat, have been gaining weight or carry your weight in the middle, your levels of insulin and the various gut peptides that regulate appetite may be turned up so high that you *think* you're hungry when you're *not*. Moreover, if you're preoccupied with thoughts of food, you'll stimulate changes in some of these levels, again mimicking hunger when your body does not need food. If any of these comments sound like yours, taking some time to prepare your body to lose weight will be essential for balanced eating to be effective:

When I eat too much at night, I'm still feeling starved the next morning.

I eat breakfast and it turns on my hunger. I'm hungry again by 10:00 A.M.

I'm always thinking about food and always feel hungry.

I never really feel very hungry but I eat anyway.

I weigh more now than I did a year ago.

How do we reset our hunger signals so that they're more accurate, so that we can relax and trust them? There are specific strategies. One is to keep busy enough so your mind is off food. Another is to exercise at least thirty minutes every day. A third is to eat less than you are accustomed to eating.

If you're not ready right now to eat less, exercise more or keep busy, don't worry about it. Come back to this process of resetting your hunger cues at another time. Be sure not to force yourself to make these changes. Forcing ourselves to eat in a certain way suggests that our food and our weight are *more important than we are*. In essence, we are denying ourselves in favor of changing one of our characteristics. This elicits the emotional stirrings of such dynamics as abandonment, rejection and servitude all rolled into one. Our predictable unconscious reaction is that the hostile, self-pitying, depressed or rebellious side of us will take over the controls of our appetite.

Many people prefer to reset their hunger signals by having a structured plan to eat less. If you're one of those people, turn to the balanced eating meals at the end of this book. Choose among those meals—or meals like them—for breakfast, lunch and dinner. If you're hungry between meals, have vegetables rather than fruit or other foods. If you prefer a less structured approach, good rules of thumb are to eat about a third less food than is your norm and consume at least five cups of vegetables a day.

After a week, your appetite regulation will be more on target and your hunger cues will more accurately reflect your body's actual need for food. At that point, you are ready to implement with success the three parts of the balanced eating cycle: eating regular meals, responding to hunger cues and eating healthy and pleasurable food.

The Balanced Eating Cycle, Part 1
Am I eating regularly?

Eating regularly means taking in food throughout the day with predictable intervals of time in between. Breakfast, lunch and dinner, just as mother always said. It doesn't mean eating by a time clock, but it does mean giving our bodies energy and nutrition on a regular basis.

If you've been eating too frequently or skipping meals, it will take some adjustments to establish a new pattern of hunger. If you aren't hungry during mealtime, eat just a little, snack a couple of hours later, and by the next meal you should be hungry enough to eat a normal meal. If you're hungry between meals, wait fifteen minutes and see if you're still hungry. The desire for food might have been triggered by thinking about food when you are bored or upset.

If you're still hungry after ten minutes, use the nurturing cycle to double-check that you are really hungry, not tired, lonely, sad or frustrated. Then, if it turns out that you're truly hungry, eat. But choose foods that have little emotional payoff, such as fruits and vegetables.

Snacking on foods that have little emotional payoff

Should you snack between meals? Definitely, if you're hungry.

My children quickly learned the right answer to "Are you hungry?" when they wanted a snack. Visions of hot cocoa with marshmallows on top and homemade cookies danced in their head although their stomachs were full. They smiled angelic smiles and said, "Starved." Fortunately, I finally caught on and began to retort, "Starved for what?"

General Times for Regular Meals

Breakfast	6:00 A.M. to 8:00 A.M.
Lunch	11:30 A.M. to 1:30 P.M.
Dinner	5:30 P.M. to 7:30 P.M.

What will *your* meal schedule be?

Breakfast_____to_____   Lunch_____to_____

Dinner_____to_____

When the choices for snacks were something crisp from the veggie bowl in the fridge or sweet from the fruit bowl on the counter, amazingly their hunger shriveled.

To make it easier to eat snacks only when hungry, consider limiting your snacks to foods with little emotional payoff. What foods skimp on comforting? You already know, but behind your personal experience is a biochemical reason. High-carbohydrate snacks—breads, cookies, milk, candies and such—boost brain tryptophan, which triggers increases in the neurotransmitter serotonin, which in turn calms, relaxes and soothes us—an emotional payoff. Fatty snacks, like potato chips and fries, don't increase serotonin levels, but they're likely to be converted into body fat. Fortunately, fruits and vegetables neither have a psychological payoff nor promote the laying down of fat. One type of sugar that is in fruit, fructose, doesn't increase tryptophan and serotonin levels, and although vegetables contain carbohydrates, the amount is so low that the emotional rewards of munching carrots, celery and cucumbers are minor.

An additional benefit of eating fruits and vegetables for snacks is that they're high in fiber and satisfy with fewer calories. Plus they vary a lot in energy content, so you can tailor your snack to fit your appetite. For example, fruits like bananas, grapes and watermelon have twice the energy of strawberries, peaches and most vegetables. When you're a little hungry between meals, a carrot or peach will satisfy you. When your appetite is more robust, a pear or a cluster of grapes is needed to take away your hunger.

By snacking this way, you won't constantly have in the back of your mind the question "Should I get something to eat?" This helps liberate you from that grating food preoccupation and allows you to give your full attention between meals to building a life that is gratifying—gratifying enough to compete favorably with a sumptuous meal or a glorious dessert.

The Balanced Eating Cycle, Part 2

Am I eating only when I am hungry?

People who have solved their weight problem don't eat much less junk food, fried food or goodies than the rest of us. The difference is that instead of eating because of food's effect as a mood elevator, calmer and distracter, they eat only when they're hungry. Moreover, their drive is not to be sure they get *enough* food, but to be sure to avoid the sequelae of having *too much*: tightness in the waist, frank indigestion and physical lethargy.

The second part of balanced eating involves honoring our bodies by obeying their signals of hunger and satisfaction. As long as you have prepared your body for weight loss by exercising, keeping busy and eating less, obeying these internal cues of hunger and satisfaction is the most accurate way to determine how much you should eat.

And you need this skill, because your body's needs vary widely from day to day and even moment to moment. For instance, a woman needs 200 to 500 more calories a day during the second half of her menstrual cycle than during the first, the equivalent of an entire additional meal. A person with a desk job during the week who becomes a tennis court warrior on weekends may need an additional 800 calories on those days. Not to mention our psychological needs—needs that separate times when an ice cream cone doesn't matter from times when it's all that does matter.

The skill of being sensitive and responsive to our hunger signals is at the heart of balanced eating. Of all the forces that detract from our ability to obey our hunger signals, emotions are the most potent. They easily overpower our biological drives. Why are they so powerful? Mainly because of the nature of emotions.

Feelings come in clusters. They are like the fabulous job that gives you a great salary and title but poor benefits and difficult co-workers. You either take the whole package of feelings or none at all. Hunger is a feeling—which is infiltrated by your other feelings. When you take your first bite of food, a flood of feelings is unleashed—not only hunger but a surge of other emotions. Both body hunger and emotional hungers are aroused by the food.

If our backlog of emotional trash is high and the stresses of the day are more than our skills in the six cures can balance, our emotional hungers will prevail, and we keep on eating even though our body hunger is telling us to stop. It's not that we don't have those body signals, but that in a shouting match between emotional hunger and body hunger, emotional hungers always win. We stop eating only when we can't eat any more, when the food is all gone or when we've eaten as much as social constraints will allow.

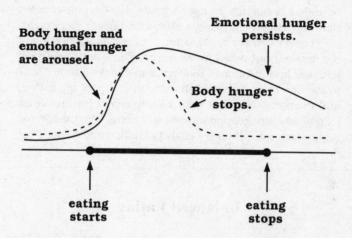

Unbalanced Eating

Body hunger and emotional hunger are aroused.

Emotional hunger persists.

Body hunger stops.

eating
starts

eating
stops

Without emotional balance, when we start to eat,
both feelings of body hunger and emotional hunger
are aroused. Our emotional hunger overrides our
body hunger and we overeat.

For some time it has been a core part of weight-loss programs
to teach people how to obey their body hunger. You may have tried
it yourself, but if you're like most of us, you found it difficult to do.
Now things will be different. With the emotional protection the
cures give you and less distress inside because of the journals
and letters you have written, fewer feelings will follow you to the
table. You will be able to hear your body's hunger signals more
clearly.

In the chart below you can see the difference. That same first
bite arouses body and emotional hungers, but now those powerful emotional hungers stay at a low level. That allows us to
become more sensitive to our body's messages after each bite, so

we can more readily pinpoint when our body hunger has faded and stop. The result is that we don't overeat.

Carl quieted the hungers that stress had aroused.

Carl was not aware when he started the program that he didn't honor his hunger signals. He later discovered that honoring them made a huge difference in his weight.

"I never saw my rapid, intense eating as a reflection of my tension, but now I know it was. The more I wrote my journals and the more I allowed people to get a little closer to me, the more I noticed that the intensity of my eating, and the overeating that went with it, were inescapable as long as my stress appetite was so strong. What made me realize this was when it began to change and I could eat

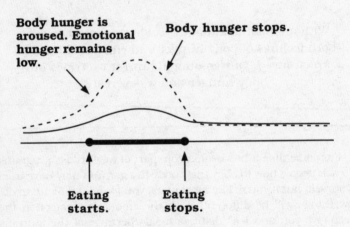

Balanced Eating

Body hunger is aroused. Emotional hunger remains low.

Body hunger stops.

Eating starts.

Eating stops.

With inner balance, the emotions that are aroused when we begin to eat are less intense. We respond to our body's hunger signals and don't overeat.

slowly and stop when I was satisfied. That's when I realized how overriding my stress appetite had been. I had been following it, rather than my body's signals."

Then he learned to read his body's hunger signals.

Carl had to learn what hunger felt like, not just anybody's hunger, but his own. He told the group that sometimes he felt cold, thought about it and realized it was because he had missed a meal and was hungry. Other times he noticed that his thinking was fuzzy, another sign that he needed to eat.

When Carl's body hunger was satisfied, he rarely stopped. What arose was the fear that he wasn't going to get enough—almost a scarcity panic. Moreover, he worked so hard during the day that in the evenings food had become his one reliable solace. He needed that emotional sustenance so much that any inkling that his food would be limited made him anxious.

Carl's weight fell quickly when his emotional appetite began to subside because of his progress in mastering the method and his "relabeling" of his hunger sensations:

"I used to think hunger was weakness and pain. I don't see it that way anymore. Hunger feels light to me and I feel thinner when I have a little edge of hunger. I don't have to run to get some food every time I get a twinge of hunger.

"The same's true for feeling satisfied. I still feel a little deprived because I want a food orgasm, or that's what I call it. I want to push ahead and totally satisfy myself with the food. What keeps me from doing that is that I've learned to hate feeling stuffed. I feel fat and I can't move. I'm more concerned these days with trying to prevent those feelings of being stuffed than I am worried about getting enough food."

How do we know how hungry we are?

Everyone is different. Your task is to watch for your own unique hunger and satisfaction signals. They're as individual as your thumbprint. When my dad becomes hungry, his stomach itches. When my son John is hungry, every emotion is magnified, and when I get hungry, I can't think!

Hunger Signals

If you are . . .

| very hungry | hungry | satisfied | full | very full |

start eating   *stop eating*

Start eating when you are very hungry or hungry.
Stop when you are just satisfied, not full.
Wait 10 minutes and you will feel full.

Feeling satisfied is even more subtle than hunger. It's the moment when all the signs of hunger are gone, yet signs of fullness have not yet begun. Here are some common signs:

- *Hungry*: weakness, irritability, tiredness, difficulty concentrating, an empty feeling, stomach sensations, cold hands or feet when the room is warm

- *Satisfied*: absence of either hunger or fullness, peacefulness, a sense of control, physical energy, loss of interest in food, emerging interest in other things

- *Full*: feeling bloated, less interest in eating, a stomachache, feeling lethargic

By using the signs of hunger and answering the questions of the nurturing cycle, you will develop an understanding of your particular hunger cues. Some of us may have difficulty recognizing these signs because of genetic factors that aren't currently well understood. Those of you in this situation will need to rely more on external signals, such as how much food you think is *reasonable* to eat for *your* body *at that time*.

The bottom line in evaluating hunger: Weight loss

How can you be sure that you are obeying your hunger signals? Weight loss. Eating for health without dieting and deprivation usually results in a weight loss that averages a pound a week. Of course if you are weight lifting, eating salty foods or, for women, around the times of menses, the number on the scale will not be an accurate reflection of your change in body fat. Otherwise, it probably will.

Katherine, a small woman with an energy level that exhausted those around her, had recently developed a weight problem. She had begun taking estrogen replacement therapy the year before and added another ten pounds to her small frame. Although changes in estrogen and progesterone do affect appetite and metabolism for some people, that wasn't the crux of the problem.

Her speedy metabolic rate had always allowed her to eat whatever she wanted without gaining weight, so Katherine was used to eating when she wasn't hungry and stopping when she was full. To compound the problem, she carried her fat low on her body where it is not as accessible to be metabolized.

The answer for Katherine was to become more sensitive to her inner signals—and obey them. In time, she accepted the essential pain of experiencing hunger now and then, and began to lose weight.

The Balanced Eating Cycle, Part 3

Is my food both healthy and pleasurable?

One day before her retirement, Marna Cohen, a cherubic social worker at the university who consulted in our eating disorders clinic, heaved a sigh and said to me, "I just listened to a 14-year-old girl agonize over how many leaves of lettuce she'd eaten the day before. It's so sad. Food is one of life's pleasures. It's meant to be enjoyed."

Marna was right. There is such pleasure in a sumptuous meal: fresh pasta with a sauce of sun-dried tomato pesto, pink salmon and extra virgin olive oil, a Caesar salad topped with shavings of Parmesan cheese, a long loaf of extra-sour French bread with a dark, crackly crust and plenty of butter—all complemented by a very dry Chardonnay and candlelight; then, for dessert, apple pie with a mound of rich vanilla bean ice cream.

How gratifying. How sensuous. How medicating. *Medicating?*

Food is one of the chief sources of gratification in life, but it is also the most powerful way we chemically regulate our bodies, and even, to some extent, our thoughts and emotions. If we fail to recognize the power of food chemicals, we give up much of our power over our own health.

George made so many good choices . . .

Remember George, the advertising executive who came to the method in "good health," only to find that the "good life" he was ingesting was negatively affecting both his health and his life? It didn't matter why he was eating that way—to please his wife, Barbara, by appreciating her robust and rich cooking, to reward himself for a hard day of work or to continue the tradition of big family dinners. All that really mattered to his brain, visceral organs, long bones and body fat was the chemical impact of his eating.

In a sense, did it really matter? Was food really that harmful? Of course not.

Food isn't toxic or even deleterious unless it's eaten to excess, but since George was cut off from his inner strength, wisdom and goodness, he ate to excess. The lull of the second drink often seduced him into a second helping of dinner. He ended the evening, not with an intimate conversation, a brisk workout at the gym or a sensual, loving interlude. Instead, he watched a little television with a bloated stomach in a depressed mood. He then went to sleep without a hint of closeness, a tad more of fitness or any sensual fireworks.

Moreover, George often awoke the next morning with a "food hangover": puffy eyes, a bloated stomach, his blood pressure on the high side and another few globules of cholesterol plaque in his arteries. And his weight certainly hadn't cascaded downward.

This man was very astute in many of his choices throughout the day—the business deal, the favor for a friend and the care with which he drove his car. But he missed a good measure of the fulfillment and success life has to offer because of the choices he made in one arena of his life: eating.

Bodies have no compassion.

What's important to remember is that bodies have no compassion. Your body doesn't care *why* you ate the food, how you *feel* about the food or what your *intentions* were. What matters to your body is what you do—what concoction of food chemicals you pour into yourself. The message is that what you eat does matter, and as nurturing as it is to eat tasty food, it is not nurturing to overeat. So, as essential as it is to avoid a sense of deprivation, it is also essential to eat foods that provide our bodies with their full measure of health.

Nancy Adler, a psychology professor at the university, gave a research methods seminar for new faculty members many years ago. One of the overriding principles, in her view, was to start with the *optimal* research design, then make the concessions and alterations that reality requires.

Similarly, you will first discover the *optimal* pattern of eating for *health* and then learn how to adapt and shift it in various directions so that your individual needs for *pleasure* will be fully met.

This doesn't answer the question "What should I eat to be healthy?" Fortunately, the same pattern of eating is optimal for losing weight, bolstering health and preventing disease. It is the nutrition of balanced eating.

The best level of fat in the diet

The fat level you choose for your day-to-day eating affects not only your weight loss but also your health. It is one factor that enhances your body's ability to prevent diseases such as high blood pressure, diabetes, heart disease and stroke.

Both the National Cancer Institute and the American Heart Association recommend a diet in which fat provides 30 percent or less of the calories. Although this is lower than the American's average intake, it may be too high for those who are overweight or at high risk of these diseases.

The Nutrition of Balanced Eating

- **15% to 25% of calories from fat**
- **15% to 25% of calories from protein**
- **50% to 70% of calories from carbohydrates, mainly from unrefined carbohydrates**
- **Adequate in vitamins, minerals, trace nutrients and fiber**
- **Abundant in the phytochemicals that prevent disease**

Heart disease is the number one cause of death in older Americans. Even though most of us have assumed that a diet of 30 percent fat protects us from heart disease, it neither regresses nor arrests this condition. In fact, a diet that is 30 percent fat allows heart disease to *progress* and the plaque in our arteries to continue to build and sets the stage for a heart attack or stroke.

Extremely low-fat diets, on the other hand, with only 10 percent of calories from fat, appear to *reverse* heart disease and might at first glance appear to be the obvious choice. Yet this level may be too low for some people. For most of us that extra margin of pleasure from a dab of butter or splash of salad dressing makes for a way of eating we can stick with.

The best level of fat in the diet for weight loss is as low as possible without creating feelings of deprivation, for several reasons.

Fat is high in calories.

All fat, regardless of kind, contains 9 calories per gram, whereas protein and carbohydrates contain only 4. So changing the type of fat you eat won't make it easier to lose weight.

Polyunsaturated fats like vegetable oils boost cancer risk. Saturated fats like those in meats and tropical oils add to the risk of heart disease. Though the monounsaturated fats in olive and canola oil don't add to the risk of either cancer or heart disease, they do pump up your risk of staying overweight.

It tastes too good to stop.

It's not that you can't enjoy high-fat foods as part of your diet, but few people can stop at small amounts of very fatty food—for instance, at one forkful of prime rib.

The *hedonic value*—a term used to describe how pleasurable a food is—is off the chart when it comes to fat. Fat is so seductively delicious to many people that they eat a whole steak even though they feel stuffed afterward.

The price we pay for our love affair with fat is high. For instance, each extra forkful of prime rib has the same amount of calories as:

- 10 cups of lettuce
- 2 glasses of milk
- 1 cup of beans
- 1 slice of grilled fish
- 1 handful of jelly beans

Fat cells are efficient at storing food fat.

The body burns only 2 percent of the fat calories we eat in the process of digesting and assimilating the fat. But it burns as much as 25 percent of the calories from carbohydrates and proteins.

If we have a weight problem, we store fat *even more* readily because we have increased levels of the fat-storing enzyme lipoprotein lipase, which transfers food fat from the bloodstream to the fat cells.

A diet that is very low in fat but stops short of being depriving gets 15 to 25 percent of its calories from fat. This is the ultimate meeting point of taste and nutrition and is the basis for balanced eating.

Please pass the sugar—in moderation.

Optimal eating for health and weight loss is based on carbohydrates—*the unrefined ones* in particular, which are low in calories, high in volume and fiber and low in fat. These include whole wheat bread, fruits, vegetables and beans. However, these may not consistently meet all your pleasure needs.

When you need a pure shot of food pleasure, what can you eat to get that pleasure while minimizing the effect of that indulgence on your health and weight?

Let's be specific. You're in a convenience store with an over-powering urge for something that tastes really good. An apple or banana would never do. Which would be the better choice—a package of sugary hard candy or a fat-filled chocolate bar?

The sugary hard candy. Yet recent research brings up some controversy about even that. A recent international symposium held in London focused on just this issue. It concluded, among other things, that both sugar and fat lead to weight gain. One study of particular interest was conducted by Danish researchers Astrup and Raben. They asked subjects to eat freely—with no restrictions on amounts—of either (1) a high-fat diet, (2) a high-sugar diet, or (3) a diet high in complex carbohydrate and fiber. What they found was that it didn't matter whether the diet was high in sugar or fat—both groups retained nearly a pound per week more than the subjects eating the complex carbohydrate diet.

This is a particularly important study because eating freely is what occurs in the real world, so it accounts not only for the impact of food on our bodies but the ways we change our eating due to psychological factors. The introduction of nonfat, high-sugar cookies, cakes and pastries kicked off a decade when obesity rates skyrocketed.

For some of us, sugar is a problem biologically.

The truth is that different people handle sugar differently. Those of us who carry our weight in the middle may be less efficient at burning up sugary foods. We may do better keeping sugar intake low. Otherwise all that sugar piles up in the blood, pumps up insulin levels and may lead the body to deposit more fat.

On the other hand, for those who carry their weight low on their bodies, a little jolt of sugar may stave off overeating. What's important is to keep amounts moderate—one handful of animal crackers, not two—and to go for sweets that are *low in fat*, such as nonfat yogurt, graham crackers or Life Savers.

For others, sugar may stimulate emotional eating.

Yet for some of us, eating sugar awakens our emotional appetite and sets our eating off and running. Once our emotional appetite kicks in, it may or may not relent after the first handful of cookies. We run the risk of a nosedive into an eating escapade and an unnecessary low. If we don't rely on the nurturing and limits cycles to restore our emotional balance, a prolonged period may result in which we romance sweets and abuse food. As a result, that first bite of a sweet may end up as more extra weight on our bodies.

So enjoy sweets in moderation. When you decide that you *really need* to have a treat, and that *the essential pain* of choosing a healthier alternative is too great, take pleasure in eating the sweet. Life is short.

Sufficient in protein

Balanced eating provides plenty of protein to meet your body's needs to build and maintain body tissues. Most women need an estimated 50 grams per day of protein, men about 63 grams per day. Balanced eating supplies about 70 to 80 grams of protein, which allows plenty of margin for those of us who have higher than average protein requirements.

Should you consume more protein than this? Probably not, but some of us could use a little more. Eating protein at a meal can keep your blood sugar up longer, staving off the midmorning craving for a bagel or the afternoon yearning to hit the vending machine. Furthermore, protein is not efficiently metabolized—you lose some of the calories in digesting and assimilating it. In addition, if you carry your weight in the middle or high on your body, having a little more protein in the diet usually results in less carbohydrate. That translates into lower insulin levels and less fat storage.

If some extra protein is good, is a lot of extra protein better? No! There are risks to a very high-protein diet. It can put stress on the kidneys to dispose of the excess protein and cause calcium to leach out of the bones and be excreted from the body, thereby increasing the risk of osteoporosis.

Moreover, very high-protein diets—even those that are low in fat—may contain as much as 1,000 mg of cholesterol, more than three times the recommended maximum. Finally, the calories consumed as protein crowd out consumption of fruits, vegetables and whole grains, which are high in substances that protect us against certain forms of cancer. As a result, eating moderate amounts of protein is the best solution.

High in fiber, a natural appetite suppressant

There is nothing quite like San Francisco sourdough bread, crusty on the outside and firm and tangy in the middle. Although its chief ingredient is white flour, so what? Eating sourdough bread is one of life's pleasures.

Yet a slice of white bread contains only 2 grams of fiber, whereas a slice of 100 percent whole wheat bread rewards us with a full 8 grams. It's as if there were two sides of a coin when it comes to food: foods that have fiber and those that don't. You can see that for yourself:

- Have some beans in a burrito? You just gave yourself a full 5 grams of fiber. But if you choose a cheese burrito instead, that number drops to zero.

- What about white pasta? It has only 2 grams of fiber. But if you order spinach or whole wheat pasta instead, you'll get 11 grams.

Why do we need fiber? There are two families of fiber and they have different effects.

One kind of fiber *dissolves in water*—pectins, gums, mucilages and hemicelluloses. They form a gel that lowers serum cholesterol about 10 to 15 percent, even if we eat only the amount per day that's in two apples or half a cup of beans. Fiber binds to bile acids, which contain cholesterol. That means the body has to take cholesterol from the blood to replenish the supply of bile acids. Moreover, bacteria in the colon make this fiber into substances that discourage the body from synthesizing cholesterol. Soluble fiber is plentiful in oatmeal, beans, apples and berries.

The second kind, fiber that *doesn't dissolve in water,* is made up of cellulose and hemicelluloses. It is found in whole wheat, such as 100 percent whole wheat bread, wheat bran and bran cereals, with lesser amounts in the cell walls of vegetables.

Insoluble fiber is a good laxative, and also seems to protect against hemorrhoids, diverticulosis and diseases of the colon, including cancer.

These are the health reasons for eating fiber-rich foods—having the 100 percent whole wheat bread instead of that fluffy white roll. Eating more fiber also makes losing weight easier. It slows down digestion, so our blood sugar stays higher for a longer period of time on the same number of calories. Moreover, fiber blunts the blood sugar peak that can lead to extra body fat in people with insulin resistance. Perhaps most important, fiber fills us up so we need to eat fewer calories to feel satisfied.

Most American adults only get a third of the 20 to 30 grams of fiber recommended by the National Cancer Institute, but we can be sure to get all we need by opting most of the time for unrefined foods, such as legumes as a vegetarian alternate to poultry or meats, whole raw fruit rather than fruit juices, and 100 percent whole grain breads and cereals.

Rich in vitamins, minerals and trace nutrients

As an undergraduate at Berkeley, I'd already found the answer to nutrition. For me, the most efficient and pleasurable way to eat well was to pop a high-potency vitamin-mineral tablet in the morning, then eat whatever I wanted for the rest of the day.

My favorite morning stop was the King Pin Doughnut Shop on Telegraph Avenue, with tall red Naugahyde stools and an elderly baker who looked like the powdered sugar doughnuts he made, dressed in a crisp white uniform with a bold tuft of snowy hair. Dinner was with the fifty other women I lived with, and we regularly gorged on batter-fried shrimp, soggy French fries and apple pie.

Unfortunately, the vitamin pill and unlimited eating idea didn't work. We can pack into pills the basic nutrients needed to survive, but if we want to live long and well, we are best served by eating a variety of real foods. This is because foods are complex amalgams of thousands and thousands of compounds.

Although it's good insurance to pop a vitamin-mineral pill every day that provides at least 100 percent of the Daily Value, that's not enough. There are more than seventy known nutrients as well as other substances foods provide that pills don't. To be optimally nourished—looking and feeling our best—takes eating a variety of foods with complementary nutritional attributes. That is precisely what is built into balanced eating.

Abundant in health enhancers

Any health food store in your town is stocked to the rafters with bottles of pills that are purported to have near-magical effects on health. Some of them do and some of them don't.

In fact, there is a whole category of substances—called phyto-chemicals—that a growing number of studies conducted in Japan and the United States suggest actually enhances health. The problem is that more and more of this research concludes that taking these health enhancers as pills doesn't produce the same boost to our health as eating them in real food. In this method, the phytochemical shot in the arm you will receive is through food.

Most of these health enhancers sound familiar—beta carotene, vitamin C and omega-3 fatty acids. Others are less familiar—including phytosterols, lycopene and isoflavones. These substances can be found in foods, particularly in vegetables, fruits, beans, whole grains and fish. A list of the common health enhancers and the light foods that are rich in them is on pages 289–92.

- "When I order a sandwich, I ask for 100 percent whole wheat bread—to get my health enhancers."

- "Yesterday I made myself a big salad. On top I put a slice of grilled fish as if it were a bonus. I was getting my health boost, just by having the fish."

"So what do I eat?"

You already know how to count fat grams, calories and per-haps check for grams of refined sugars. You learned the four food groups system in second grade and see the food pyramid on every cereal box you buy. *So what is there to learn?*

Plenty. Fortunately, most of what there is to learn involves how to use the information you already know. You need a simple system for making food decisions that won't require you to use a calculator or cause you to give up in frustration, saying, "Enough! I'll just go back to eating whatever I want."

The Solution food system is scientifically valid and *very, very easy.* All you do is eat the foods you like in each group and keep the number of servings at or above the number recommended to ensure you receive enough protein, vitamins, minerals and trace nutrients. That number is five servings each from the grain and vegetable/fruit groups and two servings each from the milk and protein groups.

The system is based on food ingredients.

The Solution food system is based on the ingredients in foods. In a sense, it's black and white. Foods are either light and thus appear on the list, or they aren't light and they don't appear on the list. When you eat for health, simply eat the foods on the list that you most enjoy. If you don't *like* celery, don't *eat* celery.

There are four groups of light foods. All light foods listed meet the criteria for a combination of factors important to health, including fat, sugar, fiber and nutrition (protein, vitamins, minerals and phytochemicals).

Light fruits and vegetables

Fruits and vegetables without added sugar or fat. Choose fresh, frozen, canned in juice or dried fruits. When you choose less processed fruits and vegetables, such as oranges rather than orange juice, your body receives more fiber. Dark green and yellow fruits and vegetables give you higher levels of phytochemicals in your diet.

Light grains

All breads, cereals and grains that contain 4 grams of fat or less per serving and no more than 8 grams of refined carbohydrates. If you choose whole grain foods, your body receives more fiber, more vitamins and minerals (especially vitamin E, selenium and zinc) and more phytochemicals.

Light milk foods

All milk products that contain 4 grams of fat or less per serving. Most of these foods are nonfat or low-fat. For instance, 1 percent milk meets the criteria for a light food whereas 2 percent milk is too high in fat to qualify.

Light proteins

All fish, poultry breasts and drumsticks (without the skin), beans, lentils, peas and meats with less than 4 grams of fat per serving. Vegetarian protein foods such as veggie burgers, tofu and tempeh are also included. When you choose fish, you give your body high levels of phytochemicals, and when you select beans, peas or lentils you boost your intake of both phytochemicals and fiber.

Now you are aware of how to eat for health: eat regularly; start when hungry and stop when satisfied, not full; and choose healthy foods you enjoy. Our next step is to balance that wealth of healthy eating with the richness of pure food pleasure.

Eating for pleasure—an essential skill

Whenever I bring up the topic of eating for pleasure in our groups, I am always met with the same response: "You mean you're telling us we have to learn how to overeat? I thought we already had that down pat. That's the reason we're here!"

There is a difference. If we are cut off from the internal wisdom, strength and goodness inside ourselves, and food has become an external solution to our distress, then overeating will add to our size.

However, once we have lessened our distress so that going inside is soothing and comforting, we can eat the "wrong" foods in the "wrong" amounts *safely.* We don't need to eat to excess that often, because there is more balance within us. Moreover, because we have a personal pipeline to our inner life, we're naturally more responsive to our body's needs. We may overeat at a restaurant and find we aren't that hungry for breakfast the next day, so we'll have one piece of toast, not two. At lunch we'll opt for a salad rather than a sandwich, not because we *should*, but because that's what we *want.* Our eating balances the overeating from the evening before, and we don't put on weight.

Furthermore, when we do eat to excess, we don't *worry* about it. There is no longer that sense of being divided—shaking our fingers at the "bad" part of us that overate. Instead we shrug with empathy and compassion and say to ourselves:

"Oh, there I go again, having too much to eat. Oh, well, sometimes I do that."

Balanced Eating *for Health*

Enjoy at least 5 servings per day of:

Light Fruits

apples	grapes	pears
apricots	kiwis	pineapple
bananas	mangoes	plums
blackberries	melons	raspberries
blueberries	nectarines	strawberries
cantaloupe	oranges	tangelos
cherries	papaya	tangerines
grapefruit	peaches	watermelon

and/or
Light Vegetables

artichokes	eggplant	potatoes
asparagus	green beans	sprouts
broccoli	green onions	summer squash
Brussels sprouts	leafy greens	sweet potatoes
cabbage	leeks	tomatoes
carrots	lettuce	tomato juice
celery	mushrooms	vegetable juice
corn	onions	winter squash
cucumbers	peppers	zucchini

And at least 2 servings per day of:

Light Milk Foods
Foods with 4 or fewer fat grams per serving:

1% milk	nonfat milk
low-fat cheese	fat-free cheese
low-fat ricotta	fat-free ricotta
low-fat yogurt	nonfat yogurt
1% cottage cheese	fat-free cottage cheese
nonfat cream cheese	lactose-reduced 1% milk
low-fat soy milk	1% buttermilk

Balanced Eating *for Health*

Enjoy at least 5 servings per day of:

Light Grains

All 100% whole grain, low-fat foods such as:
   whole wheat breads, rolls and bagels
   rye or mixed grain breads
   whole wheat pita bread
   whole wheat tortillas
   whole grain and bran cereals and oatmeal
   whole wheat pasta and brown rice
   wheat bran and wheat germ
Low-fat foods made with wheat flour, such as:
   white or flavored breads, rolls, pita bread and bagels
   French bread, rolls and bread sticks
   English muffins and crumpets
   matzoh and low-fat crackers
   white and flavored pastas
   unsweetened cereals, hot cereal and fat-free cereal bars
   pancakes and waffles
   low-fat corn or fruit breads and low-fat muffins
Other low-fat grains, such as:
   white or wild rice, corn and wheat tortillas
   millet, farina, quinoa, barley, grits, polenta and bulgur
   low-fat popcorn, pretzels, rice cakes and fat-free chips

And at least 2 servings per day of:

Light Proteins

Foods with 4 or fewer grams of fat per serving:
   fish, shellfish, turkey breast, chicken breast
   beans such as: pinto, black, red, kidney, chick peas, no-fat
      refried beans, lentils, and split peas
   low-fat lunch meats: beef, ham, chicken and turkey
   beef round, veal cutlets, skinless drumsticks, pork
      tenderloin, low-fat frozen entrees, low-fat meat substitutes
   low-fat tofu, egg substitutes, egg whites, and tempeh

"There are worse things, and I'm getting better and better at nurturing and setting limits, so I don't need to overeat as often."

All that acceptance makes those excesses less beguiling and more of a nuisance. We effectively move ourselves out of the child role in which our pleasurable eating can become excessive.

Intentional eating for pleasure is neither careless nor unconscious.

Eating for pleasure alone can be either balanced or unbalanced. Eating for pleasure in an unbalanced way is:

- Eating the sausage because it comes with the pancake breakfast even though you don't particularly want or need it

- Snacking on chips at a party or doughnuts at the office just because they're there

- Eating a salad drenched in dressing because the server didn't listen when you asked for the dressing on the side

Since what we eat has such a substantial impact on our health and happiness, this apathy, inertia and passivity is the antithesis of your weight solution. It's a way of saying "I don't matter."

Eating for pleasure alone—in a balanced way—is *intentional.* It is never passive, unconscious or unaware, and there is no guilt afterward. Eating for pure pleasure is an act of honoring yourself, not abusing or neglecting yourself, and this is why:

- You eat only for pure pleasure—without regard to the amount you eat or what you eat—when it is clear to you that you really need that food and that the essential pain of not having it is too great for you.

- You overeat in amounts or in the kind of food only to the extent that it is your need to do so, and no more. If you really *need* only half a candy bar, you throw the other half away. If you need a treat, and the *essential pain* of having frozen yogurt rather than premium ice cream is not too great for you, then you have the yogurt. Like an adult rather than a reckless, needy, hostile or depressed child,

Balanced Eating *for Pleasure*

Eat only the foods you enjoy.
Choose light foods unless you *need* heavier foods.
Choose heavy foods actively—not passively,
after using the nurturing and limits cycles, or
simply by asking yourself:

"Do I really *need* this food?"
and
**"Is the *essential pain* of not having it too
difficult for me?"**

If the answer to both these questions is yes, then
by all means *have* the food and *enjoy* it!

you give yourself all that you need and know when having
more is no longer nurturing but neglecting. Adults don't
neglect themselves.

At that point, you are honoring your reality of the moment. At
that point, no matter what you eat you will be honoring yourself.

Deirdre, the robust Canadian woman who took care of
everything and everybody as an office manager, talked
about her newfound balanced eating for pleasure:

"I used to eat food just because it was there. If the staff
was going out for lunch and everybody was ordering ham-
burgers and French fries, I'd order the same thing. Often I
didn't want that much food, but I never gave it much
thought and considered the big lunch a treat for myself.
I'm close to a weight solution now, and my eating is very
different without much fuss.

"Well, there is some fuss, and that's because I don't
go along with the crowd anymore. When we go out to
lunch I journey inside and decide what I need for lunch,

not what I'm expected to have. I eat less that way, but when I really want something heavier I have it. Yesterday, instead of eating a hamburger like the rest, I ordered a salad with nonfat dressing (I carry some in my purse), and then I had a small chocolate sundae for dessert. I really wanted it, and as it turned out, I didn't eat it all, but what I did eat satisfied me more than a hamburger would have."

Before Deirdre used *The Diet-Free Solution,* she would never have allowed herself a chocolate sundae at a restaurant. It was too decadent, and besides, what would her co-workers say when she ordered a sundae after talking about losing weight? Yet Deirdre had stopped putting others before herself and was committed to getting her need for food pleasure met regardless of the views of others. She had moved from the childish stance of wanting attention, being self-conscious and trying to please others to taking responsibility for her own happiness and pleasing herself.

There are no good foods; there are no bad foods.

Deirdre had been involved with commercial weight-loss programs for so long that she believed food was either good or bad. Although the foods that lead to optimal health and weight loss are clear-cut, *what you should eat is not.*

For instance, eating one intensely rich piece of chocolate may bring you precisely the deep sense of pleasure and satisfaction you need at the moment. In that case, eating a small piece of chocolate is far more respectful of yourself than eating the same number of calories in a lighter food—such as rice cakes. If you ate the rice cakes, you'd end up feeling both bloated and deprived. These feelings are causes of weight problems, not solutions to them.

Most food decisions are not black and white but gray. Salad with no dressing or nonfat dressing is a light food. Add one splash of oily dressing and it's heavier. Add another splash and the fat content approaches that of a pizza. It's in the subtleties between light and heavy foods that we find the balance of both health and pleasure.

Where you draw the line, in adding salad dressing, for instance, is an internal decision, one that you can rely on the nurturing and limits cycles to answer. Do you really *need* to have fatty dressing on your salad? Is the *essential pain* of having fat-free or no dressing too great?

Most evenings the nonfat dressings may meet your needs. On other evenings, a splash of oily dressing may be just what you need. Since the decisions are internal and variable, you need to check your inner life when deciding what to eat. This will enable you to eat as healthfully as possible without denying yourself the pleasure you need.

In general, *never* eat a food you don't enjoy. There are so many light foods that bring intense pleasure: ripe strawberries, a crisp red apple, a hearty bowl of bean soup with corn bread, a fresh bagel with nonfat cream cheese, barbecued salmon, baked potatoes . . . and so on. Out of deference to your health and happiness, routinely choose the light foods you enjoy.

It's a shame to eat a slab of fresh strawberry pie covered in a mound of whipped cream when you're out of emotional balance. Whether you're on a false high, an unnecessary low or simply numb, you will lack the inner balance to fully savor what you are eating.

That's why it's so essential to bring yourself back to emotional balance *before* you begin to eat. When you are in emotional balance, you're more sensitive to your body hunger and can stop before you overeat, but more important, being in balance allows you to flat-out enjoy every morsel of food!

To return to inner balance before deciding what to eat or during eating, use the nurturing and limits cycles. If you prefer, use the shortcuts to these cycles by asking yourself these questions: "Do I *really need* this heavier food?" and "Is the *essential pain* of not having it too great for me?"

If the answer to both these questions is yes, then by all means have the heavier food and enjoy it! Afterward, view the situation not as a failure but as a success. You honored your need at the time. You don't need to be perfect or to act perfectly to solve your weight problem. Doing the best you can is more than enough.

You will find that by checking in with your needs and being aware of the essential pain, it will become easier and easier to eat in a healthy way without feeling at all deprived. So your willingness to use this process, regardless of what you end up eating, is a step toward your ultimate weight solution.

Making requests of others in order to meet your food needs

Whether you want a larger dollop of whipped cream on your hot fudge sundae, or only a speck of salad dressing on your salad, you should have your food the way you want it.

This requires making requests, an essential element in balanced eating. Many of those requests will be very straightforward, such as "Please put the dressing on the side," or "Please don't put mayonnaise on my sandwich." Others are of a more sensitive nature and require more attention to the delivery. For those more delicate issues, using the hamburger sandwich technique for making effective requests is often helpful.

When I first met Anne and Kevin, the couple who resolved their weight problem together, they had major battles about where to go for dinner, what foods to keep in the house and, more important, which ones to keep out of the house. Finally, Kevin approached Anne and made a request using this technique.

The white bread: "Anne, I know we have differences about food. You want sweets in the house and I don't. It's important to me that your needs be met, but I need the food that's in the house to be right for me too."

The meat: "I feel really mad at myself after I eat the candy you have in the kitchen. I need the candy not to be in the house. Would you please talk with me and work out some sort of compromise that meets both of our needs?"

The white bread: "I know you feel strongly about this and I appreciate that you're willing to talk it through with me."

Anne and Kevin did have their discussion and both of them stayed in assertion, using "*I feel. . . ,*" "*I need . . .*" and "*Would you please. . . .*" They agreed that if Anne brought candy into the house, she wouldn't put it in their shared space. Since Kevin wouldn't know where the candy was, he wouldn't be tempted to eat it.

When it's too close for comfort, rely on the tool of the hamburger sandwich.

Discussions like these with those close to us are not always composed. They may lead to aggressive behavior, because food and weight changes can be inherently threatening.

Your strongest weapon is emotional balance. When approaching a potentially inflammatory discussion, take an inner journey in which you allow yourself ample time to regain your balance. Then, as you begin to talk with this person, vigilantly continue your inner journey, remaining aware of your feelings and needs and simply stating them.

The power behind this tool is intimacy. When you take that extra millisecond to preface your request with the words *"I feel . . ."* you create an intimate connection rarely encountered in day-to-day life.

It can be disarming to others because they would feel much more reassured if you acted disconnected, not intimate, and passive or aggressive rather than assertive. If you were to act passive, aggressive or removed, that behavior they know how to handle.

But if you act assertive and engaged, they must stop and deal with themselves and you. They will find it unsettling and even embarrassing to continue to act childish when you're acting like an adult. What's more, they're frightened because indirectly you're asking them to join you above the separation of the generations line. They know that if they refuse, they look foolish in their own eyes and in yours. Moreover, it's not easy to bully or hide from people who are clearly balanced in their own inner life, empathetic toward yours and doing nothing more than stating their feelings and needs.

In fact, healthiness is catching. Often the assertion, balance and connection you offer have such a powerful effect that your adversary takes your hand and joins you above the line. The advantages to you are that the request you have made is more likely to be met, and perhaps more important, in a world that dishes up alienation, treachery and isolation, you have created a moment of intimacy.

Asserting Your Food Needs

The white bread
(honest compassion)
"I understand that you eat differently."
"I care that this affects you."
"It matters to me that this will work for you."

The meat
(a clear message)
"*I feel* angry when you bring junk food home.
I need you to keep it out of the house for a month.
Would you please do that?"

"*I feel* frustrated that we eat so late.
I need to eat by 7:00 P.M.
Would you please talk with me about making
some changes?"

"*I feel* afraid that if I cook heavy foods for you,
I'll eat them.
I need half our family dinners to be healthy.
Would you please make this change?"

The white bread
(honest compassion)
"I appreciate that you will do this."
"I know it isn't easy."
"Thank you for supporting me in this way."

You can stay in the adult role
even though they don't.

Let's say things don't go well. At that moment this person is
not capable or willing to cross the line and assume an adult role.
They remain passive, aggressive or removed, but you still have
your power. Even if they remain in the child role, you can continue to stay above the line, facing the essential pain of this per-

son's current state, rechecking your feelings and identifying your evolving needs.

The essential pain in this case may be that you can't have what you want right now. Your job is to not abandon yourself, but continue using the nurturing and limits cycles until you have regained your inner balance. For instance, when the essential pain is that you can't have what you want from this person right now, you may become aware of a wide range of feelings and then formulate needs that respond to them:

- *How do I feel?* A little disappointed, perhaps. *What do I need?* To back off for now and ask again later. It's not that important.

- *How do I feel?* Angry. *What do I need?* To make another request, to be certain this person understands how important this is to me.

- *How do I feel?* Depressed. *What do I need?* To check my limits because my thinking may be powerless and negative and my expectations may be too low.

- *How do I feel?* Furious. Enraged. Hostile. *What do I need?* To check my limits. Perhaps my expectations are too high. Maybe I'm not facing the essential pain that this person has separate and important needs, too.

Again, the answers are not what matters. What does matter is that you keep asking yourself the questions of the nurturing and limits cycle until you restore your inner balance. Then, even if your need is not met over the food or other issue at hand, you haven't lost the war, because you have maintained your inner balance and had the personal dignity to stay in the adult role.

What lifestyle surgery do you need?

The *lifestyle surgery* for the balanced eating cure involves making changes in your food environment that will foster balanced eating in your life.

The goal is to adjust your food environment so that it's easier to eat in a balanced way. Although these external limits are not substitutes for internal ones, they are extra tools you can use to resolve your weight problem.

"I need to keep all the ice cream and cookies out of the house."

"I need to shop for fruits and vegetables during the week."

"I need to keep a bag of apples in the trunk of my car."

"I need to have dinner earlier."

"No more Sunday-morning pastries."

Give yourself whatever lifestyle surgery you need. Many of these external changes will be temporary. You will need fewer and fewer of these external limits as you near your weight solution. However, do not judge yourself if you need external limits on food forever. The decision that set those limits was an *internal* one. It's not as if the diet Gestapo or nutrition police locked up your refrigerator. You decided for yourself that you needed those external limits. You knew and accepted yourself enough to make the changes you needed in your food environment as a way of ensuring your success. Bravo!

There are no nutritional cliffs to fall off.

In the end, after endless diets and food facts, the balanced approach to eating, the one that resolves weight problems, turns out to be neither rigid nor demanding. There is no nutritional cliff to fall off if you eat a little too much of this or that.

We can relax and approach our eating in a balanced way with reverence for our bodies. We can eat healthy foods while still allowing ourselves a measure of lust when we need to experience food's pleasures and the comfort of feeling full.

As you can now see, The Solution gives you personal license to be completely free to meet the food needs of your body, mind and spirit. You know that it is ultimately up to you alone to bring yourself the vitality, pleasure and comfort you need from food.

You don't have to *control* yourself any longer.

What is most gratifying and a tremendous relief as well is that you don't have to *control* yourself any longer. There is an immense security in knowing that nothing *terrible* will happen. You can unleash yourself to eat freely and still find, time and time again, that your eating remains relatively balanced.

This occurs not because you are perfect, but because you have accepted how delightfully *imperfect* you are. At some instant, through the journals, the letters or life's revelations, you were able to show yourself compassion and accept your dark side. You bravely confronted yourself and asked if those flawed parts of yourself were friend or foe. With grace in your heart you reached out and embraced . . . the friend.

From this new perspective, you became fully aware of your inner balance. Food became just food. The clamor from your past about how much of this or that to eat began to sound rather silly. You could soothe yourself from within and comfort yourself with the strength, wisdom and goodness that was always inside you but was only now fully apparent. And as you did, you found that balanced eating wasn't so difficult after all.

Cure 6. Mastery Living

At a recent, admittedly boisterous group session, I asked every-one, "If you were to construct a day for yourself that truly met your needs, what would it be like?"

Joanne smiled, "Winning the lottery, making love all night and dancing until dawn."

George said, "I'd unplug the phone, get take-out food and watch old videos."

Cure 6. Mastery Living

An active and fulfilling lifestyle

3. Time to Restore

1. Exercise

2. Meaningful Activities

What would *you* say? Perhaps something similar. Yet a steady diet of life's peak experiences probably wouldn't satisfy us in the long term any more than we'd be satisfied with a colorless life of few pleasures other than food.

Despite our individual differences, there is a style of living with universal appeal, one that responds to the basic needs common to us all: to move, to work and to restore. It is called *mastery living*.

Mastery living focuses on the day, making it complete.

In mastery living, each day becomes a separate entity that is complete in its own way. Each day we move our bodies, engage in meaningful activities and restore ourselves—not just with sleep, but to regain our balance physically, emotionally, intellectually and spiritually. Life's focus shifts away from the pursuit of some perfect future or the payoff of immediate gratification at all costs.

George Leonard, in his classic book *Mastery*, asks us to honor the "in-between" days, to take as much pleasure in them as we do in the peak times. According to Leonard, "The achievement of goals is important. But the real juice of life, whether it be sweet or bitter, is to be found not nearly so much in the product of our efforts as in the process of living itself, in how it feels to be alive."

It's a paradox, but those who reap the richest rewards from life *and the most success* seem to do so by valuing the journey, not the result. This journey—the master's journey—involves being willing to attend to the covert process of learning, even when overt progress is not apparent. A life of mastery living is devoted to the balance we find in the present. If we focus on the pursuit of a future goal and lose that balance, "a large part of it may well be spent in restless, distracted, ultimately self-destructive attempts to escape," according to Leonard.

In the long run, if we push to achieve some future goal and lose our balance in today, reaching the goal is tinged with bitter memories, and we must return to life to pick up the pieces that were broken on the way. It is neither pleasant nor efficient.

By the same token, the pattern of seeking immediate reward undermines our success as well. There are few shortcuts in life, and when we delude ourselves that there are, we end up disappointed with the results. We neither achieve our goal nor reap the desired rewards.

We already have a good foundation to achieve mastery living.

Applying these concepts to your weight solution turns your attention from appreciating only the climactic moments—the paid-off mortgage, the happy, successful adult children and the achievement of a career—to finding the rhythm and grace of the day.

Marsha always thought she achieved at work.

Marsha supervised a large staff at the university and was a stately professional woman who seemed quite polished and composed. The only source of disappointment in her life was her weight, which had seesawed up and down thirty pounds several times in the past decade.

Marsha saw her weight as the price she paid for success. Yet embedded in her weight problem was a lifestyle that not only contributed to her weight difficulties, but held her back from achieving even more professional success.

At first Marsha discounted the idea that driving herself too hard not only increased her weight but made her less productive at work. In fact, her first reaction to mastery living was, "I could never do that. I push for the goal and don't protect myself from the work it takes to get there."

"I can tolerate focusing on the day . . . "

Later, her views began to shift. "I'm beginning to think that I can tolerate focusing on the day, but it's still so difficult for me. The part of me that has to have my way and have it now can't tolerate living with so much lack of resolution." The door had opened just a crack—enough for her to entertain the idea of investing in mastery living.

The next few weeks in Marsha's life were a metamorphosis. She submitted to the three parts of mastery living, taking an hour walk at noon, questioning what activities had meaning to her and giving herself ample time to restore herself each day. She shared with the group, "I have given up control. I'm only holding myself accountable for the day, not the project. I'm trying to make each moment and each day have some balance."

Marsha already looked different—the first sign that she had embraced mastery living. However, it wasn't yet the size of her body I noticed, but the relief on her face and how her shoulders lost their stiffness. She was finally relaxed.

Having a longer fuse and losing weight

Within a few weeks Marsha saw two of the bottomline results of mastery living: a weight loss and a change in her work life. "Now that I'm committed to living in a balanced way, I notice that my fuse is longer. I don't pop off at my staff as much. I used to feel guilty after we met a deadline. The sense of achievement was always tarnished by memories of some of the things that were said and done to meet that deadline.

"Now I seem to be able to keep it together during the rough times, so there are fewer hard feelings afterward. There's a different tone in our office now, probably because there's a different tone in me."

Shifting our time horizon and filling universal needs

You may not live like this now. Few people in the Western world do. Yet in pursuit of solving your weight problem forever, consider making small shifts in your lifestyle so that your needs— which are universal—will be met. As you move your body daily, take time for activities that have meaning and allot time and attention to restoring yourself, your weight will gravitate to a level within your genetic comfort zone.

This is a time to keep an open mind. This cure makes no rigid demands, because there are hundreds of ways to weave exercise, meaningful activities and restoring time into your day. However, the key to making mastery living a way of life rather than a temporary experiment is *fluidity*. It is your ability to move and change with your interests, situations and needs.

Mastery Living

Exercise:	30 to 90 minutes each day of *physical activity*
Meaningful Activity:	time each day for pursuits that *you find meaningful*
Time to Restore:	activities that restore you physically, emotionally, intellectually and spiritually

Author Carlos Castaneda told the story of Don Juan, the sorcerer. In *Journey to Ixtlan*, he urged that we free ourselves from daily routines that dull perception, and the past itself, which is imprisoning. He said, "Nobody knows who I am or what I do. Not even I. . . . We either take everything for sure and real, or we don't. If we follow the first path, we get bored to death with ourselves and the world. If we follow the second and erase personal history, we create a fog around us, a very exciting and mysterious state."

Although the fog might not entice you, the reality is that your needs are fluid. One day you're in a running routine that you love; the next day you turn your ankle and are out of commission for a week. *What do you do?* For a while yoga classes bring you a certain peacefulness and strength. Then your favorite yoga instructor, whose voice soothes and rocks you, moves to Alaska, and her replacement reminds you more of a drill sergeant. *What then?*

Security comes from developing a consistent responsiveness to the present. By letting go of *what was, what ought to be* or *what will be*, you prevent your mind from getting in the way of your heart. You can then construct an evolving lifestyle that offers precisely the movement, meaning and restoring required to meet your present and ever-changing needs.

It doesn't matter what you do, only that you do *something* that meets your needs for fitness, meaning and restoring yourself. The ultimate yardstick for each part of this cure is nothing that anyone can see. It is your answers to internal questions:

- Do I feel physically fit—that is, strong in wind, solid in muscle and supple in flexibility?

- Does my day have meaning? Am I doing things that draw me away from myself and calm me down because I know that what I'm doing matters?

- Do I generally feel restored at some point during the day: that is, are my needs—physical, emotional, intellectual and spiritual—being reasonably well met?

If you can respond affirmatively to most of these questions most of the time, then you have achieved mastery living.

The Mastery Living Cycle, Part 1

Am I physically active?

I remember years ago being an anxious young faculty member who rushed out to read and absorb every new study on exercise that hit the journals. Somewhere along the line, I stopped rushing.

As nice as it is to know that the thermic impact of exercise differs between those who are overweight and those who are lean, or to recognize that it takes twenty-five minutes of biking and only fifteen minutes of running for physical activity to have an aerobic effect, these facts are not the answer to incorporating physical activity into the daily routine to produce optimal fitness.

The answer is to move. Therefore the first part of the mastery living cycle is quite simple. Exercise daily for thirty to ninety minutes.

Moving your body every day . . .

Studies have shown that regular physical activity is the best predictor of keeping weight off once it's lost. For example, Ewbank and colleagues reported in 1995 that in a sample of 45 people who had lost weight two years before, the more active the subjects were, the more weight loss they maintained.

The minimum amount of exercise recommended by the College of Sports Medicine and the Centers for Disease Control and Prevention is thirty minutes of moderate-intensity exercise for most of the days of the week. This recommendation is not based on what people do, but on what their bodies need. Only about 22 percent of Americans actually are that active.

You may have expected them to recommend less exercise because you've heard that cardiovascular fitness improves if you exercise three times a week. You're not exercising for cardiovascular fitness alone, however, but for other reasons, including weight loss.

Not only does more time spent exercising burn more energy—those extra few bites of dinner are released as heat rather than sequestered as body fat—but activity brings increased feelings of well-being and relaxation that guard against a rampant appetite.

According to Kevin, "I have no choice but to exercise after work. If I come home and eat, it's nutritional suicide. If I work out first, I'm not so hungry and I'm not so pent up. I can eat a sane meal and be satisfied."

With all these benefits—burning calories, revving up your metabolism, lifting your mood, dissolving stress and a calorie-free way to satisfy emotional appetites—moving your body each day is one cornerstone of mastery living. Exercising the body becomes as important a part of the daily routine as brushing your teeth or taking a shower. It's something you do preventively to stay clean and fit and balanced on the inside.

How much is too much?

What about a maximum amount of daily exercise? Isn't more better? Frankly, no, for several reasons.

For one, overexercising is associated with increased injuries to muscle, bone and tendons. Moreover, several studies show that at very high levels, overexercise is associated with increased mortality. A study of nearly 17,000 Harvard alumni found that the beneficial impact on longevity of moderate levels of exercise vanished as moderation turned to excess. Another study by Steven Blair found a slight increase in death rates from all causes among women who were engaging in the heaviest workouts.

Overactivity can detract from health and inner balance.

I have seen countless patients overexercise in a way that detracts rather than adds to their health.

Often the second run of the day or the third hour at the gym does not fulfill a physical purpose, but an emotional one. Overactivity can be a smokescreen for not having mastered the other cures. In such cases, our real power is to master those cures, not cover them over with excessive activity.

Marty's emotional overeating crept back now and then, and she complained to me about it. Her opportunity was to use the symptom of emotional overeating to remind her to take inner journeys more often, use the nurturing and limits cycle and quiet her drives to overeat.

However, Marty had given the journals and the letters only a quick once-over because she was reluctant to feel the discomfort that occurs before pent-up feelings are released. As a result, it was still difficult for her to take inner journeys as often as she needed them to keep in balance.

Marty wanted to continue to lose weight, so she gravitated toward more exercise, until she was going to the gym twice each day and playing women's soccer three times a week. She had no time left to restore herself and explore meaningful activities.

It was only when she cut back on her exercise activity that she had the focus to journey inside, relieve her emotional distress and return more often to inner balance and natural—rather than forced—weight loss.

Low versus high intensity

Total body fitness requires activities that foster endurance, strength and flexibility. Endurance is the most important because endurance activities that use the large muscle groups in continuous motion burn up calories and improve cardiovascular fitness. Strength-building activities are also important for the boost in muscle mass that increases the body's caloric need. Flexibility activities increase range of motion, decrease risk of injury and improve performance of day-to-day activities as well as various sports.

Low-intensity endurance exercise like walking, biking or exercising on a treadmill is ideal if you have not been active recently. In time, as you become more and more fit, you can extend the period of your exercise and add some other activities—for "cross-training"—that are slightly more intense or offer the added benefits of strength or flexibility.

You may have heard various arguments for low- versus high-intensity exercise. Most discussions have focused on the fact that at less intense activity, a higher percentage of calories burned is fat. That's interesting information, but not the whole story.

Chester Zelasko, Ph.D., from Buffalo State College, noted that at lower activity levels the energy came half from burning carbohydrates and half from burning fat. When people exercised at somewhat higher intensities, about 70 percent of the energy came from carbohydrates and about 30 percent from fat. Even though the calories burned over forty-five minutes of exercise were higher for intense exercise (288 versus 218 calories), the amount of calories from fat was about the same.

What's difficult to determine is what to value. More people will exercise at lower intensities, and the fat loss is about the same as with higher-intensity activities. Several studies by Ewing and others concluded that it didn't matter how much fat was burned. Maintaining a weight loss was related to how much energy was expended in exercise, not how much fat was burned.

Yet the plot thickens further due to postexercise oxygen consumption, which is a fancy way of saying that after exercise people continue to burn extra calories, even if they're sitting down. Yet the average number of calories burned per workout is only 5 to 10 after low-intensity exercise, 12 to 35 after moderate exercise, but as high as 180 after higher-intensity exercise. As a result, there are some advantages, if you are already physically fit, to increasing the intensity of your workout.

Let's put these ideas together into some recommendations.

The Solution Exercise Program

The Solution exercise program categorizes activities as either basic or cross-training and involves three levels, each with more time spent in exercise.

Level 1: Basic Activities

Unless you are currently highly fit, begin with Level 1, which is thirty minutes daily of basic endurance activities, such as walk-

The Solution Exercise Program

Level 1. Begin with:

30 minutes of basic activity per day.

Level 2. When you are ready for more:

Increase the time to 45 minutes and add
cross-training activities.

Level 3. When you are ready for still more:

Increase the time for basic and cross-training
activities to as much as 90 minutes per day.

ing, treadmill or cycling. After a period of time, this amount of exercise won't be enough for walking, treadmill or cycling, but it can be any activity that is continuous, uses large muscle groups like legs and arms and lasts at least fifteen minutes.

Choose something that you *enjoy* doing that fits well into your daily life. Good examples are walking, rowing machine, biking, stationary biking, aerobics classes and jogging. The key here is enjoyment, so consider the context of your exercise: Is the physical environment pleasant? Will you do it alone for solitude or with a friend for socializing? If the plan you construct is not pleasurable enough to make you to want to do it, keep searching until you find a better plan.

What will you do for your basic daily activity?

Levels 2 and 3: Cross-Training Activities

After you have exercised at Level 1 for some time, you will be likely to notice that it is not enough. You will want or need more to give you that same postworkout sense of well-being.

That is the time to move to Level 2. At this level you will exercise forty-five minutes a day and include cross-training activities in your program. This will give you variety to meet your changing fitness level, moods, interests and schedule. Moreover, simple endurance activities won't give you all of the strength and flexibility needed for total body fitness.

To ease into the Level 2 exercise program, you could add a more intense activity to your basic one, such as jogging for a while when you would normally walk. Take up weight lifting and stretches at least a couple of days each week. Plan ahead for seasonal sports, and find activities you can do that are playful, like horseback riding, jazz dancing or soccer.

When you are ready for still more—which may take a year or two—begin Level 3 exercise and increase your basic and cross-training activities to as much as an average of ninety minutes a day.

What cross-training activities do you prefer?

"What is the right intensity of exercise for me?"

The right intensity is the one that keeps your heart rate at 12 to 15 beats for six seconds, which is between 120 and 150 beats per minute. You may occasionally add more intensity, but this is a safe and fat-burning intensity for basic exercise.

Another way to determine if you are in this safe but effective zone is to observe your breathing. When you are walking, for instance, you should be sucking air into your body involuntarily in a much more vigorous way than you would at rest, but not so much that you couldn't talk easily if you were exercising with a friend.

"How do I know if I'm overexercising?"

You know you're overexercising if you feel exhausted after exercise or the next day, if you don't feel refreshed by the time you start the next exercise session or if you notice a soreness or some pain that doesn't abate.

Most of us at this point in our fitness awakening can't get enough exercise and it's frustrating to cut back, but now is the

Cross-Training Activities

Type	Examples	Your Preferences
Intense Activity	jogging, Stairmaster, soccer, aerobics classes, skipping rope	
Strengthening Activity	weight machines, free weights, karate, home strength training routine	
Stretching Activity	yoga, home stretching routine, ballet, jazz dancing, tai chi	
Playful Activity	horseback riding, family wrestling, Rollerblading, all kinds of dancing	
Active Interests	gardening, walkathons, foot races, backpacking, mountain climbing	
Warm-Weather Sports	golf, tennis, swimming, kayaking, hiking, crew, soccer	
Cold-Weather Sports	cross-country skiing, hockey, ice skating, aerobic tapes, mall walking	

time to adopt a more relaxed approach. Admit to yourself that life is long and it's OK to cut back a little on exercise for now. The results will be enhanced fitness in the long run. You can always be flexible with yourself and switch to a less strenuous form of exercise for a day or two, like doing stretches if you are feeling achy or doing upper-body weight training if your legs are sore. As soon as you feel better, continue with your normal program.

"How do I know when I'm ready for the next level?"

Your workouts should leave you feeling physically refreshed and emotionally positive. When they stop rewarding you in these ways, and it's not because you've been overexercising, it's probably time to increase the duration of your exercise or the intensity or both. Move slowly into a new phase by gradually adding more intense or longer workouts, until you are using your new exercise routine daily.

"How do I get back on track when I'm off track?"

This is perhaps the most important question you could ask about exercise. Various studies show that once people begin to exercise they stay with it—until something disrupts their schedule. Then we find ourselves stuck in the no-exercise rut for far longer than we care to admit. Unfortunately, there is always something to disrupt our schedule:

"I was fine until I went on vacation. I haven't exercised since I got back."

"The kids were sick and I stopped going to the gym. It's hard to start again."

"This deadline at work made everything go on hold, including my exercise."

This is where your ability to journey inside pays off. It can recharge your exercise commitment, even when exercise is the *last* thing you want to do.

The Nurturing Cycle

I feel . . . guilty I haven't exercised.

I need . . . to start, but I don't want to.

Would you please . . . help me with my exercise program. I'm off track.

The Limits Cycle

I expect . . . myself to do something to get started again. Anything I'm willing to do.

I think . . . that it won't be so bad. I don't have to exercise for long, and I don't have to do things I don't want to do. I always feel better after I start exercising again. I actually enjoy exercising.

The essential pain . . . is that starting again is difficult. If I don't start now, it will only become harder to start again. What feelings does that bring up? Anger, sadness. Can I feel those feelings, face them and follow through anyway? Yes.

What about the television?

Your challenge is not only to exercise, but to enhance your general activity level. Why? Because active pursuits keep you from thinking about food and triggering your appetite mechanisms so you think you're hungry when you really aren't. Because staying involved and active adds to the calories you burn each day. And because such activity keeps you from engaging in the passive national pastimes of watching television or sitting at the computer, which make your metabolic rate plummet, as Yale's Kelly Brownell said, to "near comatose levels."

As a general rule, limit television, computer play, reading and other sedentary activities to no more than one hour at a time. Crowd them out with active interests that fit into your weekly schedule, such as gardening, golf, hiking, skating and household projects.

Avoiding aches, pains and injuries

If you are awakening to the idea that exercise is actually . . . fun, you may become so excited about being strong, supple and sturdy that you overexercise and lay yourself up with an injury.

We're all vulnerable to injuries when we're on the path to becoming fit, especially if we're on the heavy side. So it's even more important for us to check our bodies for aches and pains and, if necessary, switch to forms of exercise that will give those body parts a rest. Also, early on in your march toward total body fitness, stay away from sports that have ballistic movements— that is, cause you to extend your body in more extreme positions—such as soccer or basketball. When you have achieved a higher level of fitness, you'll be more likely to engage in these activities without injury.

Of course, according to sports medicine author and physician James Garrick, M.D., be sure to attend to injuries early on rather than letting them mount up, whether that requires that you see a sports medicine physician or a physical therapist or just endure a few ice packs and get some rest.

The Mastery Living Cycle, Part 2

Am I engaging in meaningful activities?

Mastery living involves striking a balance between ourselves and others—that is, shaping a lifestyle that takes care of ourselves, but not *only* ourselves. It is the careful balance we strike between feeding ourselves and feeding others that brings us fulfillment.

David Sheppard Surrenda, Ph.D., explained it to me this way: "Life is an anxious experience. Much of food and other problems are responses to trying to cope with the intensity of feeling life, as if we're saying: 'This is too intense. Let me eat.' In fact, we often run from the tumult of life by doing something soothing that numbs those feelings."

Meaningful pursuits melt the tension, soothe the anxiety.

If exercise relieves tension, meaningful pursuits melt it away. Of course, when pursued to such an extreme that we neglect our responsibilities and needs, meaningful activities become external solutions. However, in moderation, they are sublime because they relieve us of the burden of being self-absorbed.

Does that mean that you must save starving children in Ghana to lose weight? No.

Meaningful pursuits exist by the million. And most are in your own backyard. Perhaps you need to "bloom where you are planted"—and find more meaning in your current work and play. On the other hand, a little lifestyle surgery may be just what you most need. If so, you can modify your lifestyle to add a few more activities that you view as meaningful.

Stanley finds meaning in basketball and gardening.

Stanley, the physician, had been burdened with a preoccupation with weight and food since childhood. As he focused on meaningful activities, he realized that his work was so emotionally taxing it was no wonder he collapsed into the routine of television and dinner in the evenings.

What he needed more than anything was a meaningful activity that had nothing to do with sick and dying patients. What that turned out to be for Stanley was two things: spending time playing basketball with neighborhood teens who didn't have dads around, and gardening. He began a fern garden on his deck, and inside he devoted a room to growing bonsai plants. When he arrived home from work, his solace wasn't food, it was quietly tending to his plants and playing a little basketball.

Two very different approaches . . .

Recently, watching one woman in a supposedly tedious, vacuous job made me appreciate the option of making the work you do meaningful in its own way.

Near my home in a large mall is a small airline ticket office where I was picking up a ticket for my father. In the course of the long delays and frustrating mix-ups, I noticed how differently the two airline representatives, one a man of substantial size and the other a rather lean woman, both in their early fifties, approached their work.

Their jobs were tedious, in an office that could be crammed with impatient customers one hour and completely empty the next. I noticed that the woman—her name tag said Stella—went out of her way with every customer she served, not only to see to their needs, but to make them feel special and cared for. When the quiet times came she pulled out a magazine, in a directed fashion, and read it with intense interest. Stella seemed to find meaning in her work, and appeared quite balanced and fulfilled.

On the other hand, the man, Roger, who was helping me, seemed distracted and anxious. It was as if he was just barely managing to tolerate me, his job and himself.

Moreover, Roger disappeared every few moments to the office behind the counter. Each time he reappeared, he was chewing and swallowing and looking guilty as if he was doing something he just *had to do*, but *knew he shouldn't*. Because his work appeared to hold little meaning, Roger *needed* that food. Except that his need wasn't for food—he needed a way to take the edge off the burden of self-absorption and relieve the anxiety of being alive.

Which meaningful activities will you weave into your life?

It was cultural. Everybody had boring jobs and big appetites.

Anne's story was very different. Anne lived in a family that was accustomed to a lifestyle of work, dinner and television, as were most of the families in their neighborhood. What was meaningful about her parents' work was that it kept the electric bill paid and put groceries in the cupboards. It kept the family going.

As an adult, Anne kept up a similar lifestyle, and it wasn't a problem for her except when her weight crept up and her blood pressure was on the rise:

"I never thought our family pattern of routine work, excessive meals and numbing out with television was anything but normal. Meaningful activity for my family was just getting through the day. Were they satisfied and ful-

Meaningful Activities

Friends
I made a point of calling a friend who was upset.
I invited a friend to take a walk with me.

Partner
I shared an intimate moment with my spouse.
I went out of my way to be kind to my partner.

Family
I taught my child something today.
My mother was sick and I called her to cheer her up.

Community
I am part of my church community.
I go to the town meetings and keep involved.

World
I am active in environmental issues.
I keep up on world affairs.

Work
I take pride in doing a good job at work.
My work helps people and has meaning.

Money
I am paying my bills and saving for retirement.
I donate to the causes I care about.

Home
I fix things around the house.
I take pride in making a warm and orderly home.

filled? I don't think so, or there wouldn't have been so much blatant overeating. But in all honesty, I don't think my parents even thought about whether or not they were happy. They accepted life as it was."

And who really knows for sure whether or not Anne's parents found their work meaningful enough to remove them from life's anxieties? Only they would know, because the very nature of meaningful activities is that it doesn't matter what they are. It only matters that they have enough meaning to the individual to coax that person away from life's harshest emotions.

For instance, it doesn't matter if you wash windows or watch your child's soccer team. If those activities take you out of yourself and supply you with a sense of meaning, purpose or altruism, then that's enough.

Although I've listed a few examples of activities that are meaningful to others, your challenge is to find those that are *the right fit* for you. Some of the activities you decide on may require some lifestyle surgery—that is, structural changes in your life—like leaving work early or going back to school. Others will simply evolve in the context of your current activities, just as Stella took pride in not only doing a job well, but doing it with an appreciation that both she and others mattered.

The Mastery Living Cycle, Part 3

Have I restored myself?

Part of the fallout of seeking external solutions—whether they be food or activities—is that we run the danger of depleting ourselves. When we fall victim to the illusion of unlimited personal energy, we end up sliding into the pit of exhaustion.

My father has always coached me, "Pace yourself." I can't say I've always followed that advice, nor, coincidentally, has he. When he gardens he digs like crazy all day instead of stopping and resting. Neither of us is dealing with reality when we don't take time to restore ourselves. *We're acting like kids.* Instead of taking responsibility for putting quarters in our meter all day, we run on the false high of unlimited personal energy, only to slide later on into an unnecessary low of exhaustion.

Fortunately, using the nurturing and limits cycle brings out the reasonable side of us that slows us down long enough to replenish ourselves.

The Nurturing Cycle

I feel . . . depressed and exhausted. Useless. Frustrated.

I need . . . to stop overdoing so much. To take time to restore myself.

Would you please . . . talk with me as I plan some changes. On my own I seem to continue in the same patterns.

The Limits Cycle

I expect . . . to be able to do all the things I want to do. I expect to have no end to my energy. Is that a reasonable expectation? No. What is a reasonable expectation? To do the high-priority things and let the others go. Or take longer to get things done. Not to work straight through, but take breaks to restore myself.

I think . . . that if I don't get it done now, I never will get it done. If I don't do everything, I'll end up doing nothing. Is that helping? No. What would be positive and powerful? To say to myself that it's the quality of the journey that counts. To focus on what I'm doing now and doing it well. To find balance and completeness in the day. That is where my success lies.

The essential pain . . . is that I can't do everything I want to do. That I have limits. That I'll die without having done all the things I want to do. What feelings come up when I face that fact? Sadness. A lot of sadness. Is it going away? No, not yet . . . yes, it's fading. I feel back in balance. I will expect less and focus on the balance of my day more.

What restores us is as individual as our thumbprints.

What you do to restore yourself is strictly a matter of your own particular needs.

For most of us, time to restore incorporates a mix of rest, emotional sustenance, intellectual challenge and spiritual fulfillment. Perhaps the most abstract of these is emotional sustenance, which typically involves emotional intimacy, personal pleasure and sexual satisfaction.

Emotional intimacy naturally flows from the nurturing cycle because you have mastered the skill of connecting with yourself and can more readily connect with others. The limits cycle helps you shift your boundary from thin to thick, depending upon the safety of the person you are with, so acquiring closeness is less risky. Intellectual challenges, likewise, are rather easy to come by, whether through books, tapes, classes, films or computers.

Sexual satisfaction is more elusive for some, particularly those of us with weight issues. Velia Frost, M.S.W., explained this to me years ago: "The most primitive expression of sexuality is oral. It is *eating*. It is *food*. So unless sexual needs are met, our gastronomic appetites speak to us in a multitude of erotic tones, all of which miraculously blend into the single word *more*."

Which activities will you use to restore yourself?

Your sexuality belongs to you.

One might also say that sexuality is something you possess apart from your partner. A priest, Tom Allender, teaches that human sexuality is an expression of your essence. It belongs to you to enjoy and to attend to, whether or not you are involved in a physically intimate relationship. It is your responsibility.

People possess their own sexuality, as the arousal occurs *within* them. We are the keepers of our sexual satisfaction. Just the way it's our job to be sure the grass is cut or the children driven to school, it is our task to attend to meeting our sexual needs.

Many of us with weight problems have less sexual satisfaction than we would like. It may be that we've turned off sexually altogether and wonder if we even have a libido, or that we don't make love often enough or with enough passion and pleasure. Perhaps we have sex too often, somewhat indiscriminately and in ways that fall short of pleasuring.

As a result, our oral needs for food may increase. Some of us may eat more in an indirect attempt to satisfy our libido, which may further wane. For others, an increase in our weight results in our being less sexually alert and sensual. We neglect our own responsibility to our sexual fulfillment, and we may not even know we are doing it.

Assuming responsibility for meeting our sexual needs—even if they seem muffled by time, habit and health—may mean any-

Restoring Activities

Body

sleeping	relaxation	sexual pleasure	back rubs	nice clothes
resting	massage	a new haircut	foot rubs	being hugged
grooming	baths	a new style	sleeping in	holding hands
sensual activities	stretching	adornments	soft blankets	a long shower

Mind

reading	adventures	Feelings Letters	listening	journal writing
learning	writing	a new interest	talking	dreaming
creating	time alone	gardening	cooking	fixing things
reflecting	yoga	being outdoors	cleaning	phoning a friend

Spirit

meditation	art	dance	poetry	prayer
singing	crying	laughing	intimacy	inspiring reading
nature	music	community	animals	journal writing

thing from developing one's skill at self-pleasuring and engaging in sensual activities alone or with another, to seeking counseling for an issue that hampers your fulfillment with your partner.

Perhaps it means getting a baby-sitter, working a little less or gaining more body pride. Meeting this challenge is often formidable for those with a history of abuse or who use weight to say no to sexual advances. But the extent of the challenge doesn't shrink the need. A degree of sexual fulfillment remains important to accomplishing mastery living, personal balance and a weight solution.

Which restoring activities do you need more of?

Most of us have at least a few areas in which our lifestyle falls short of restoring us:

"I just need some sleep. I need to go to bed by 10:00 P.M."

"I'm lonely. I need more time with close friends. In fact, I need more friends."

"I'm bored. I need more intellectual stimulation. I need to learn something new."

"I feel alienated from my community. I need to become more involved."

"I'd like to make love more often and be more romantic with my mate."

How can we possibly take time to restore ourselves when there *is* no time? The job, the commute, the kids, the partner, the friends, the bills, the exercise routine and meaningful activities virtually cram the day with activity. There's no time left for refueling.

Rearranging the outside to make it easier.

You may well need to do some *lifestyle surgery* to rearrange your life so that you will have time to restore yourself, and for physical activity and meaningful activities as well. Making concrete changes lends structure and support to our personal decision to make our lives better. Here are some common forms of lifestyle surgery that pave the way to achieving mastery living:

"There's no way I can commute four hours a day and have time for a balanced life. I need to work closer to home."

"I can't work through lunch anymore. I'll have to bring workout clothes to work and take that time for exercise."

"I live in a totally chaotic relationship. There is no way I can restore myself with that turmoil in the home. I must improve the relationship or leave it."

"My heart isn't in my work. I need to find a job I can put my interest in, something that has more meaning for me."

Certainly mastery living requires rearranging priorities, activities and situations so that it's reasonably convenient to live in a balanced way. Accomplishing this shift in the texture of our day calls for goodly amounts of attention, discipline and creativity. Yet most program participants say that living each day as if it were complete in and of itself brings a whole new dimension of peace and fulfillment to their lives.

As you turn out the light in the evening . . .

When you have mastered this method, your situation is different. By journeying within, you have expressed the strength, goodness and wisdom you find inside yourself in your style of living. Imagine your life with inner balance and mastery living:

As you turn out the light most evenings, you think back over the day with a sense of completeness and a feeling of gratitude. There was dignity and security in the day because you have attended to the myriad of needs of your body, mind and spirit. You have created a life that is good after all.

Part 4
A Clear and Simple Method

Trust enough to follow the checklist.
Then watch your dreams of health and
happiness come true.

Your Own Pathway: A Checklist

There is no right or wrong way to use this book, but many of those seeking to master the method will find that the easiest and most natural pathway is to follow the steps shown on the checklist below.

It's simple enough. Start with reading Parts 1 and 2 of the book to understand the method, assessing your own weight and enhancing your skills at going inside.

Then you will read about the cures in Part 3—and you'll naturally start using them—and writing some of the journals and letters to make going inside easier. When you are ready, you will finish the rest of the journals and letters.

If you like added structure, you may decide to use the cure records—one for each cure—as a weekly support for your progress.

The unexpected rewards will begin to be yours and you will spontaneously let go of external solutions, including those related to eating and activity. Your weight will continue to decrease in a gradual way until it finds a level that is within your genetic comfort zone.

Last, you will realize that, in fact, the agony is over and you are cured.

The Solution: *Your Own Pathway*

_____ 1. Understand the method (Part 1).

_____ 2. Assess your weight (Part 2).

_____ 3. Master the skill of going inside (Part 2).

_____ 4. Begin using the cures:

- read each cure chapter (Part 3).
- write Journals 1 to 8 (Part 4).
- write 20 Letters (Part 4).

_____ 5. Finish the Journals and Letters (Part 4).

_____ 6. If needed, use the Six Records (Part 4).

_____ 7. Regain your inner balance. You will naturally let go of external solutions, eat less and exercise more.

_____ 8. Feel the joy of being cured.

The Thinking Journals

There are thoughts I don't want to think about. As luck would have it, they're precisely the ones I most need to think about. Why? Because thinking these thoughts opens up wellsprings of feelings that otherwise stay locked inside me—which is hardly productive. Because feeling and releasing these intense feelings is the ticket to regaining joy, spontaneity and exuberance.

The journals and letters move us through three stages.

The Thinking Journals and Feelings Letters work in tandem. You write a journal to bring up the precise thoughts that will be most powerful and helpful for you to think. Then you heal the feelings that arise from these thoughts with the letters.

Thinking Journals bring up the precise thoughts
we need to think in order to heal.
Feelings Letters heal the feelings those thoughts
bring up.
It is this two-step—the journals and the
letters—that help us release the past more easily.

Not only will each journal and letter shed another layer of your emotional armor, but the journals move in stages, and as they move, so do you. The three stages are:

1. healing old hurts

2. accepting ourselves today

3. shaping the future

The letters you can do alone, with a friend or with a therapist. Because these are sensitive and powerful issues, many people find that they benefit from having some kind of outside support as they write them. In fact, if you have a history of depression, hostility, emotional problems or stress-induced medical conditions, it's essential that you have the warm support of a therapist as you do these letters. Gaining this kind of guidance can move you through the stages more safely and more rapidly.

Stage 1. Healing Old Hurts

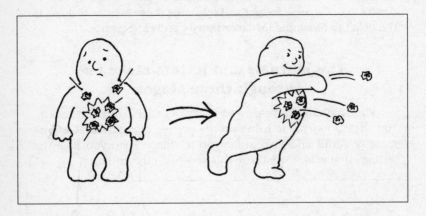

The first stage of your weight solution is having the courage to go inside yourself and examine the various pieces of your emotional distress, feeling the feelings each evokes and then releasing them. This takes courage. But it doesn't take more courage than you possess. Consider this stage with curiosity and compassion, as if to say to yourself:

"Gee, I know there's a lot of stuff in there. Guess I'd feel better if I got rid of some of it. How interesting it will be to see what comes out. After all, I'm just human. Nobody can be my age without some angers, hurts, fears and guilt.

"It will be such a relief to get some of it out in the open, so I can see it in the light of day, then release it—in other words, to give myself a good internal housecleaning."

The topics of these journals are very straightforward. You will trace the stages of developing your weight problem and the important events that surrounded them. This will guide you in understanding and healing key points in your personal legacy.

Then you will explore the six causes of weight problems because they are your particular story of the most important areas of your coming of age. You will think about the patterns in your early years, especially those with influential people in your life, such as parents.

When you have completed these first eight journals—and the letters that accompany them—you will have released so much internal distress that you will *feel* better—so much better, in fact, that you'll be ready to move above the separation of the generations line into the adult role, where your power and balance lie.

Stage 2. Accepting Ourselves Today

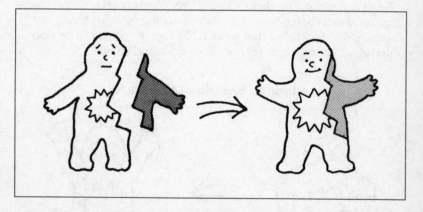

The second stage of your weight solution is a time of accepting the past and strengthening your identity. The essential shifts in our thinking that this stage requires are (1) grieving our losses, (2) realizing that we are alone and (3) accepting our dark side.

The losses to our own lives caused by not having mastered

these skills are now clear to us, and it's time to grieve those losses and go on with our lives. By feeling and releasing the emotions these losses produce, we move ourselves into emotional balance so we can progress with the developmental shift this stage heralds.

Accepting our aloneness is the next step. Carl Greenberg, who directs the behavioral medicine program at the University of Washington, confided in me one day, "The critical moment comes when a person faces that *we are all born alone and die alone.* From that point on, everything is different."

We face that moment . . . and the essential pain passes. Then we feel a surge of excitement and energy. No one will rescue us from life but us. We are the only ones who hold the keys to the doors we must open if we are to be happy and healthy. For the first time it is apparent to us that we actually do possess all the keys we need.

This awareness of the solitary nature of life catalyzes a period of deep self-reflection. If we avoid it we may fall into a depression or retreat into using external solutions. If we embrace it, we will find a new intimacy with ourselves and others.

The next step is accepting our dark side, which draws upon the more nurturing inner voice we are developing. We approach our flaws, flub-ups and weaknesses by extending to them a warm hand and casting on them a loving eye. We accept them, and this acceptance relieves us of the sense of being split between "bad" and "good." We realize that we don't have to be perfect to be wonderful. At once we cast off both arrogance and shame.

Stage 3. Shaping the Future

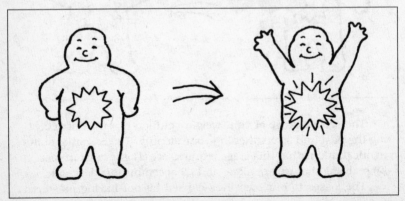

By this stage, to a greater or lesser degree, you have healed old hurts, come to terms with your aloneness and compassionately accepted your dark side. Now something inside you shifts:

"Something's changed. I don't know what it is, but it feels good."

"I don't want to go back to the way I was before, but can I do this? Can I live this way with all this energy?"

"What's strange is that I have no appetite, I mean, no big appetite. Food is just food, nothing more. I don't want to eat, I want to live!"

"All the things I've never done, I want to do!"

When the blood is coursing in our veins, and life is spelled out in neon before us, food looks rather mundane. Certainly not something worth harming health and happiness for. Now our challenge becomes nailing down that newfound aliveness and moving ourselves into a future that feels markedly different from the past.

The most effective way to own that aliveness, aside from continuing to master the six cures, is to *act* on it. In this cluster of journals you will attach words to your dreams and actually make them become real.

Sex, love and rock 'n' roll

Jim wanted what he had never had: a healthy, loving relationship where the dizzying falling-in-love stage didn't die, but evolved into a love of greater erotic pleasure and more emotional depth. A year after Jim mastered this method, not only had he kept his weight off for the first time in his life, but he had a warm, loving relationship with someone he'd met dancing.

Jim was beaming when I saw him at one of the Saturday retreats we have for graduates of the training. His words jumped out of him. "My life is transformed. I love this person, but it's not fading. Our love is just getting stronger, and I know it's that my limits are so much better and I'm able to give in a way I couldn't before, because I nurture myself better. This is what I wanted in life, to feel balanced and healthy in my own life and deeply in love in a healthy relationship."

For Alicia, what mattered was Argentina.

Alicia wanted more in life than being caught up in her work and the lives of her sisters. She started reserving energy just for herself, and began saving money for a trip to Argentina. The next time I saw Alicia, she looked vibrant, healthy and trim. Her skin was smooth and her face peaceful.

She smiled at me and pulled from her purse a tiny ceramic plate from Falafate, a small village in Argentina that she had visited. On it was a vase of blue and pink flowers, clearly in balance, with a few sprigs of leaves trailing off to the sides, fully alive.

Who says you can't dream about work?

When I first met Marian, she had started her own business, which wasn't flourishing the way she had hoped. It was only as she mastered the method that she fully appreciated who she was and wasn't—she didn't have marketing skills but did have a gift for helping people relax and feel safe learning computer software. She found a marketing consultant and her business began to turn around. More important, she looked different—not just her weight, but her enthusiasm for her own life.

Just like Jim, Alicia and Marian, you have dreams and now it's time to take them seriously. You matter and how you feel counts. Is it OK to go to Argentina? Is it reasonable to hope for a deep romantic love? Is building your own business worth doing? By all means, yes. This is *your life*, these are *your dreams*, and you have acquired for yourself the skills and courage to make them real.

Writing your journals

Your journals will be your responses to the questions that are posed. Tell the facts as you see them, plain and simple. Stick to writing about what you think rather than how you feel. If the journal topic asks you to reflect on your parents, consider your parents or others who took on the role of raising you, whether they be siblings, grandparents, stepparents or friends. As soon as you have completed your journal, express your feelings through one or more Feelings Letters.

Stage 1. Healing Old Hurts

Journal 1. *Your Weight Story*

Tell the story of your weight. In this journal please talk about any times when you gained weight and the situations, changes or stresses within one year of that time. Do this for when you first gained weight and for later times when your weight increased. Then write Feelings Letters about each of the situations, changes or stresses that occurred.

Journal 2. *The Stages*

The purpose of this journal is to recognize the developmental process, how your weight problem developed in stages. Note the points when (1) stress mounted, (2) balance was lost (going inside was no longer comforting) and (3) overeating and inactivity began. Write at least one Feelings Letter.

Journal 3. *Strong Nurturing*

Please tell the story of your nurturing. Specifically, think about your pattern of recognizing and expressing feelings and needs and making requests of others. Please describe (1) the way your parents nurtured themselves, (2) how they nurtured you, (3) the ways they taught you to nurture yourself and (4) how you have nurtured yourself during adulthood. Then write at least one Feelings Letter.

Journal 4. *Effective Limits*

Please tell the story of your limit-setting. Specifically, think about reasonable expectations, positive and powerful thinking, facing the essential pain and following through. Please describe (1) the way your parents set limits with themselves, (2) how they set limits with you, (3) how they taught you to set limits with yourself and (4) how you have set limits with yourself during adulthood. Write at least one Feelings Letter.

Journal 5. *Body Pride*

Please tell the story of your body pride. Specifically, consider weightism, using body size to express yourself and accepting and honoring your body.

Please describe (1) the body pride of your parents, (2) the body pride they showed toward you, (3) what they taught you about body pride and (4) the ways you have or have not had body pride as an adult. Write at least one letter.

Journal 6. Good Health

Please tell the story of your health. Specifically, think about your daily awareness of your body's health, vigilant self-care and effective health care. Describe (1) how your parents took care of their health, (2) the ways they attended to your health, (3) what they taught you about taking care of your own health, (4) how you've taken care of your health in your adult years. Write one or more letters.

Journal 7. Balanced Eating

Please tell the story of your eating. Specifically, consider eating regular meals, eating when hungry, stopping when just satisfied, not full, and choosing foods that are healthy and pleasurable. Describe (1) your parent's eating habits, (2) how they fed you, (3) what they taught you about eating and (4) your eating habits in adulthood. Write at least one letter.

Journal 8. Mastery Living

Please tell the story of your lifestyle, specifically, taking time each day for exercise and meaningful activities and time to restore yourself. Describe (1) how your parents lived, (2) how you lived as a child, (3) what your parents taught you about achieving a healthy, fulfilling life and (4) how you've lived in adulthood. Write at least one letter.

Stage 2. Accepting Ourselves Today
Journal 9. Facing the Loss

Please describe how not having these six skills has affected you in your adult years. Be specific. To the extent that you were not equipped with the six cures, what were the consequences to you? Write at least one letter.

Journal 10. Realizing It's Up to Us

There is no one but you who can bring you mastery of these skills now. Therefore, at this stage, that which was our parents' responsibility to teach us, we must teach ourselves. We must *bring ourselves up.* Please discuss (1) why your parents fell short of giving you the six cures and (2) what made it difficult for you to give them to yourself in adulthood. This is a very important journal. Please write a letter to each of your parents and to yourself.

Journal 11. Accepting Our Dark Side

Please describe the things about yourself that you are not proud of. Take the stance of a loving but honest observer and make a list of your flaws, faults and shortcomings. This is your dark side. Some of these characteristics are changeable; some will probably never change, so they require your understanding and even your compassionate acceptance. Write letters to each fault you listed until you stop judging your dark side and begin to feel compassion and acceptance.

Journal 12. Achieving Intimacy

With full acceptance of yourself, you're an integrated adult. You now have the composure and generosity to give and receive in intimate relationships. You can tolerate the risks of surrender and rejection and you have the limits to know when it is safe to be close to someone and when you need distance from them. Please describe (1) the ways in which intimacy has been difficult for you in the past and (2) at least one person with whom you would like more intimacy. Write one or more Feelings Letters.

Stage 3. Shaping the Future

Journal 13. Renewing Hopes

As you write these pages, suspend your logic and encourage your imagination. Allow hopes, dreams and fantasies to arise. Picture the life you want for yourself, the way you want to live and the sources of fulfillment you want to experience. Please describe them. Write one or more letters to yourself.

Journal 14. Dreams That Come True

Bring up the image of the life you want for yourself. To make that dream real, which of the six cures would you need to strengthen—nurturing, limits, body pride, good health, balanced eating or mastery living? Which of these cures are you willing to strengthen in order for your hopes to become reality? Write one or more letters to yourself.

Your Journal Checklist

Journal 1. Your Weight Story

Journal 2. The Stages

Journal 3. Strong Nurturing

Journal 4. Effective Limits

Journal 5. Body Pride

Journal 6. Good Health

Journal 7. Balanced Eating

Journal 8. Mastery Living

Journal 9. Facing the Loss

Journal 10. Realizing It's Up to Us

Journal 11. Accepting Our Dark Side

Journal 12. Achieving Intimacy

Journal 13. Renewing Our Hopes

Journal 14. Dreams That Come True

The Feelings Letters

There may be a jumble of feelings inside you because you've written a Thinking Journal or because the workday has been filled with events like spilled coffee on final reports, flat tires on the way to work or a vexing spat with a co-worker. Those feelings can spell trouble: false highs, unnecessary lows or numbness, including the numbness that comes from repetitive thoughts.

How to get out of your thoughts, into your feelings and on to healing yourself? Feelings Letters. We've used this tool for ten years with the program and it continues to get rave reviews as people use it to smooth out the bumpy road of human emotions. But before I show you how to use this five-minute technique to managing feelings, let's look at the theory behind it.

Feelings aren't alone. They come in stacks.

This technique draws on the work of John Gray, Ph.D., who first wrote about the feelings letter he developed in *What You Feel, You Can Heal*, which is among the selected readings at the end of this book.

According to Gray, feelings are "stacked up" one on top of another. Let's say you're aware of feeling angry. Chances are that you also feel other feelings but you're not aware of them. Sure, you could feel and express your anger, but that wouldn't lead back to inner balance. You'd probably still feel anxious or upset or

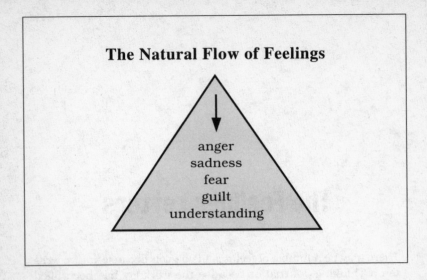

The Natural Flow of Feelings

anger
sadness
fear
guilt
understanding

stressed. Why? Because the other feelings that are stacked beneath your anger remain within you.

It's only when we can feel and express the whole range of feelings that there is healing. Only then can we feel acceptance, understanding and love. That's right. Under all those layers of difficult feelings are positive ones, and that only makes sense. Because if we didn't *care*, we wouldn't feel so distressed. When the dog chews up our brand-new boots, we feel more upset than when he destroys our worn-out running shoes. A falling-out with a close friend distresses us more than an unpleasant exchange with a stranger.

This stack of feelings can be felt and released one by one. The natural flow of feelings for many of us is anger, sadness, fear, guilt and understanding. The Feelings Letter guides you in feeling and expressing each one so that you can heal and comfort yourself.

In which feeling are you likely to become stuck?

Most of us have one or more feelings that trip us up for a long period of time. We can't seem to shake the feeling and we don't know why. The emotion feels so enormous not because it is—but because the other unexpressed feelings haven't been felt and expressed.

If this flow is not working, thoughts pile up:

A PILEUP OF THOUGHTS
repetitive, obsessive

no
feelings

If this flow is not working, we get stuck
in one feeling:

STUCK IN ONE FEELING
such as depression or hostility

The Feelings Letters help us restart the natural
flow of feelings.

What is the feeling in which you become stuck? Anger? Sadness? Fear? Guilt? Or do you find that all feelings are blocked out and all that is left is endless, repetitive thinking? In both cases the remedy is the same—to start the flow of feelings once more. And the Feelings Letter is an effective way to do that.

The Feelings Letter

The letter is addressed to a person, situation or thing that is important to you and about which you are feeling distressed. It is also used after writing a Thinking Journal. Some people write Feelings Letters routinely, such as during the time they take to restore themselves each day, before going to bed, the first thing in the morning or even at their lunch break.

None of the specifics of your pattern matters, really. All that does matter is that you write the letter and release the feelings. You address it to the person or situation that bothers, upsets or distresses you, and then one by one you feel the feelings and write them out: anger, sadness, fear, guilt and understanding. You sign the letter and add a P.S. about what you need from the person or situation and what you need from yourself.

That's it. That's all you do. It will remove another piece of distress from your inner life, and with that remarkable unloading, you'll find it easier and easier to tap into your inner life and soothe and comfort yourself from within.

Most people need at least sixty letters to clear away the emotional trash.

How many do you need to write? Start with one and commit to the process of writing the letters—even daily if you will—until you can sense relief in your inner tensions. The good feeling of relief will prevail, and the frequency of writing the letters can then subside a little.

Most people find they need to write at least sixty letters to clear away their emotional leftovers. Sounds like an effort, but it's actually a relief. Clearing all those feelings away lightens you more than losing sixty pounds. A pound per letter, that's about right. That's how Mary Lou saw it.

> "I didn't become an accountant because I was the artsy, expressive, warm type. I'm a logical, thinking-oriented person and that's how I like it. I did one Feelings Letter in the group, mainly because of social pressure. Everyone else was doing it. I was surprised to find that it really did work, in fact, remarkably so.

"I can't account for what happened after that except to say that I liked the economy of releasing these feelings more efficiently and, in a way, continuing them because once the anger was out, I knew the next feeling would come up and it would lead somewhere. It wasn't as if I worried that I would get stuck in depression and never get out.

"Sometimes I'd write a letter and it wouldn't resolve anything. I'd still have some resentment toward some people, particularly my sister, who can destroy me with a glance, or my mother, who's disappointed in me. So I'd wait a day or a week and write the letter to them again, and in time the letters have relieved me of a lot of my hurt and hostility toward them, and myself too. I wrote one letter to my appetite and another to the fat on my legs and both were big breakthroughs for me."

Start with just one letter. *Just one.* Here's how . . .

How do you write a Feelings Letter? Simple. Just write a Thinking Journal. Or if you prefer, just bring up some thoughts about something that is distressing to you, and address a letter to the person, situation or object involved.

Try to bring up feelings of anger. When they arise, begin writing and express your anger using any words you like. Write your anger without restraint, using expletives, aggressive language or anything that comes rushing out of you. After a while you'll notice that the feeling has faded.

When it does, wait a moment and notice what feeling comes up next. Sadness. Feel the sadness and then write out those feelings too. Then pause and bring up a new feeling—this time fear—and write to express it. After feeling and expressing anger, sadness and fear, it is often easier to see our contribution to the problem—that is, what we did or didn't do, felt or didn't feel, said or didn't say. If we're willing, next the guilt is felt and expressed, which is remarkably relieving.

Last, with this whole range of feelings expressed, a rush of understanding often occurs and a sense of acceptance, even love, prevails and we write it in our letter. After signing the letter, it's time to check for needs, answering the questions "What do I need from you?" and "What do I need from myself?"

You can't do this letter wrong.

Use this letter in the way that works best for you. Take as little or as much space as you need for each response in your letter, and if you come to a feeling and don't feel it, that's fine, just go on. Later you may feel it or you may not.

If you come to the end of the letter and do not feel a sense of understanding and acceptance, that's fine too, but it typically means that you didn't express enough of one or more of the feelings. Perhaps then or at another time you'll write another letter on this same topic and more of your feelings will emerge and be healed.

Ways to use your feelings letter . . .

What does one do with a Feelings Letter? Whatever is right for you. I toss some of my letters out, save some, read some to the people I addressed them to or ask one of those people to read the letter to me. It's even helpful to read one's Feelings Letter out loud alone. Anne wrote to her husband, Kevin, in the middle of the night after a quarrel:

> "I was upset. I knew I felt awful inside, so I left the room and wrote a Feelings Letter. I felt remarkably calm after that. I could see where I was being unreasonable. When I returned to the bedroom I gave him the letter. He read it, then tossed it away, furious. I felt calm. The letter had put me back in emotional balance, and a turn around the limits cycle made it clear to me that I couldn't control whether or not he was willing to talk about the problem constructively that evening.
>
> "Kevin didn't write a letter and unfortunately stayed angry and didn't sleep a wink all night, or so he told me the next morning. Yet I felt accepting of the situation and slept well for the entire night."

The Feelings Letter may or may not help Anne and Kevin resolve their differences on a particular issue, but at the very least, Anne was able to reclaim her balance, which matters. If she hadn't, she would have been up worrying all night and the happiness and health of her next day would have been compromised without any benefit to their relationship.

Marian, the woman with the entrepreneurial business in computers, wrote a Feelings Letter to her father, who raised her. Her relationship with him had always been strained, and for the last three years she hadn't seen him. Although she felt justified in keeping her distance from her dad and his critical attitude toward her, she felt sad about it. He was her father—the only father she would ever have. She wrote several letters to her dad over a period of a month.

Several months later, during the holiday season, Marian saw her father, and for the first time in many years was able to talk to him without expecting him to be perfect or having a covert agenda of punishing him. To Marian, this was a major accomplishment, and she saw a big change in her attitude.

"I feel like I've gotten some peace about my dad. Instead of carrying this hate around inside me I understand that he's an unfortunate person in many ways. I need to protect myself from him hurting me, but now I can find ways that we can enjoy each other at times. I feel like I've grown up!"

Use the following guide to help you get started with the letters and the checklist to keep track of how many you have written.

Dear Dad:

Anger *I hate it that you acted like you were so good and you weren't. You gave me what you wanted to give me: food, presents, television, not what I needed. You weren't a loving father to me, you were self-centered. I was alone and needed someone to be there for me.*

Sadness *I feel sad that I didn't have someone there who really loved me, who wanted me and thought I was wonderful.*

Fear *I'm afraid I deserved your neglect. I'm afraid there is something unlovable about me, and that I am a bad person. I'm afraid you'll never love me.*

Guilt *I feel guilty that I don't call you. I feel ashamed that I dislike you. I regret that I haven't made an effort to reconcile with you.*

Acceptance *I understand that the situation was hard for both of us and that you did the best you could.*

Signed, Marian

P.S.

What I need from you . . . *is to tell me you weren't a perfect parent and you wish you could have been there for me more.*

What I need from myself . . . *is to write these letters again until I feel more accepting of you.*

Feelings Letter

Dear _____

Anger   (I feel angry that, I can't stand it that, How could you . . .)

Sadness   (I feel disappointed that, I feel sad that, I feel unhappy that . . .)

Fear   (I fear that, I am afraid that, I feel scared that . . .)

Guilt   (I feel sorry that, I regret that, I feel guilty that . . .)

Acceptance   (I understand that, I care that, I accept that . . .)

Signed_____

P.S.

What I need from you . . .

What I need from myself . . .

Your Feelings Letters Checklist

To release the past, write Feelings Letters. Each time you write a letter, check off another number.

____ 1.   ____ 2.   ____ 3.   ____ 4.   ____ 5.

____ 6.   ____ 7.   ____ 8.   ____ 9.   ____ **10**.

____ 11.   ____ 12.   ____ 13.   ____ 14.   ____ 15.

____ 16.   ____ 17.   ____ 18.   ____ 19.   ____ **20**.

____ 21.   ____ 22.   ____ 23.   ____ 24.   ____ 25.

____ 26.   ____ 27.   ____ 28.   ____ 29.   ____ **30**.

____ 31.   ____ 32.   ____ 33.   ____ 34.   ____ 35.

____ 36.   ____ 37.   ____ 38.   ____ 39.   ____ **40**.

____ 41.   ____ 42.   ____ 43.   ____ 44.   ____ 45.

____ 46.   ____ 47.   ____ 48.   ____ 49.   ____ **50**.

____ 51.   ____ 52.   ____ 53.   ____ 54.   ____ 55.

____ 56.   ____ 57.   ____ 58.   ____ 59.   ____ **60**.

The Six Cure Records

Some people progress faster in mastering the cures when they record their use of the cures on paper. Use these cure records in any way that gives you the structure you need to move quickly in mastering the cures.

In Solution groups, participants choose one cure record per week to complete. This gives them an opportunity to plan how they will practice one specific cure, record their progress and later evaluate what they accomplished with that cure and what remains a challenge for them.

Of all the behavioral techniques that encourage people to change, recordkeeping is by far the most effective. Consider experimenting with using the cure records to give you a little added motivation and support.

Cure 1. Strong Nurturing

Notice your feelings and needs throughout the day. Meet your needs, asking for the support you require.

	Sun	Mon	Tues	Wed	Thur	Fri	Sat
My Feelings How do I feel?							
My Needs What do I need?							
My Requests Would you please . . .							
Was my need met?	yes no	yes no	yes no	yes no	yes no	yes no	yes no

Cure 2. Effective Limits

You check your expectations to be sure they are reasonable, and your thoughts to be sure they are positive and powerful. You feel and let fade the essential pain and follow through.

	Sun	Mon	Tues	Wed	Thur	Fri	Sat
My Expectations reasonable							
My Thoughts positive and powerful							
My Essential Pain feel and let fade							
Did I follow through?	yes no	yes no	yes no	yes no	yes no	yes no	yes no

Cure 3. Body Pride

You experience body pride throughout the day, avoiding weightist thoughts, using words, not weight, to express yourself and honoring and accepting your body.

	Sun	Mon	Tues	Wed	Thur	Fri	Sat
Weightist Thoughts Avoided this thought:							
Instead thought:							
Words, Not Weight Used words to express:							
Honor and Accept Showed body pride by:							
Did I feel body pride?	yes no	yes no	yes no	yes no	yes no	yes no	yes no

Cure 4. Good Health

You take care of your body, checking how it feels and what it needs and following through with self-care and health care so that you have the vitality you need to enjoy your life.

	Sun	Mon	Tues	Wed	Thur	Fri	Sat

Check My Body
The good feelings:

The difficult feelings:

Self-Care
What I did:

Health Care
What I did:

Did I feel healthy?   yes no   yes no   yes no   yes no   yes no   yes no   yes no

Cure 5. Balanced Eating

Your eating is balanced. You eat regularly throughout the day, starting when you are hungry and stopping when satisfied, not full. You eat food that is healthy yet pleasurable.

	Sun	Mon	Tues	Wed	Thur	Fri	Sat
Regular Meals							
Ate breakfast, lunch and dinner							
Responding to Hunger							
Hungry when started							
Stopped when satisfied							
Responding to Hunger							
5+ Fruits or vegetables							
5+ Grains							
2+ Protein							
2+ Milk							
Was my eating balanced?	yes no	yes no	yes no	yes no	yes no	yes no	yes no

Cure 6. Mastery Living

Your lifestyle is active, fulfilling and restoring. Each day you take time for exercise, meaningful activities and restoring yourself physically, emotionally, intellectually and spiritually.

	Sun	Mon	Tues	Wed	Thur	Fri	Sat
Exercise Daily (30+ minutes)							
Meaningful Activities Daily							
Time to Restore Daily							
A day of mastery living?	yes no	yes no	yes no	yes no	yes no	yes no	yes no

The Joy of Being Cured

The word *cure* conjures up visions of something ethereal like a magic potion and a miraculous healing. Better yet, it stirs up images of flashy instruments and penetrating lasers. *The Diet-Free Solution* is not like those cures. However, even though it's not magical, miraculous or flashy, it *is* penetrating and it *is* a cure.

The evidence comes from all sides: the research of others, our own studies, the experience of children, the track records of adults, the excitement of other health professionals and its effect in my own life.

Yet all those pieces of evidence aren't as convincing as the tone of reverence in the voices of those of my patients who have truly mastered the method. Their sentiments are stated quietly but clearly—the method has transformed their lives on levels far more abstract than the flesh that lasers touch. Its impact on their lives has spanned far more realms than the classic cure can possibly reach.

When are you cured?

When you feel balanced much of the time and
have received the six unexpected rewards.
The struggle is over, the drama has ended and
the weight problem is *gone*.

A different kind of cure

Some people experience what Suzanne did:

> "I've lost thirty-five pounds this year and I'm proud of it. I won't say I'm not. But it's the deeper changes that I cherish the most. I'm not the same person I was. I feel balanced and secure—and my life has so much more meaning and fulfillment. In fact, the whole drama about my weight—the anxiety, the embarrassment, the sense of failure—seems remote to me now. My weight problem has been cured."

Others find that the cure is more subtle. Anne was one of them. Her success was wildly apparent to others—her weight was down, and her face was radiant. Anne's vibrancy and balance were spreading out into her work, her mothering and her marriage. Yet Anne minimized her success when her negative, perfectionistic thinking periodically returned.

> "I ate some chocolate fudge cake at the party and then I had a second piece. I was so full when I was done that I felt uncomfortable. It's rare that I do that anymore, but it really bothered me. Sometimes I'm afraid I'll never be completely over my weight problem."

Eating two pieces of a cake at a party was *not* evidence that Anne had not solved her weight problem. In fact, *listen carefully* to Anne's next statement. Embedded in it is irrefutable evidence that she was, in fact, cured.

> "When I eat that way, I say to myself, 'There I am overeating again. I know I'm going to gain the weight back.' Then I use the limits cycle to protect me from myself—and I keep using the cycles until I'm back in balance."

A cure occurs when you stop abandoning yourself.

How can you tell that Anne had cured herself? Despite her disappointment about overeating, she did *not* abandon herself. In her early years there was no one who stuck with her to help her sort out her feelings and straighten out her thoughts even when she took "too long" or needed "too much."

Anne has mastered the skill of treating herself in a different way than she was treated growing up. She doesn't abandon herself but listens to her inner voice—using the tools of the method over and over again—until she returns herself to inner balance.

Yet you might say that she didn't do it *perfectly*. She ate the cake and she fell into her old pattern of negative thinking. She didn't need to do it perfectly to be perfectly cured. Life is long and there's plenty of time for her to regain her balance. And when she was ready, she did regain it.

A cure does not mean you will never gain another pound, eat too much pizza or take a break from exercise. It means that you are loyal enough to your inner life that you can regularly access the strength, wisdom and goodness within you. As a consequence, the times when you seek external solutions will be infrequent and short-lived—which means that your weight problem is solved.

You can do this too. You are capable of staying in balance.

As you stay in balance and solve your weight problem, people will watch your eating and your weight:

- Are you gaining the weight back?

- Did you really eat *that much* French bread?

- Are you *supposed* to have all that butter?

Instead of listening to them, you will laugh to yourself. So what if you gain a few pounds back? You have the tools to reconnect with your inner life when you are ready to. Their doubts, fears and jealousies are their affair anyway, not yours. You know weight is the symptom, not the problem, and the solution is not to fret about a pound or two, deny yourself French bread when you need it or scrape the butter off the baked potato when the pain of doing so is too great for you. The solution is to draw upon the power within you, which you were born with, then lost, and have now reclaimed.

You have earned the six rewards: *integration, balance, sanctuary, intimacy, vibrancy* and *spirituality*. As a result, even though the cat still howls in the night, the alarm still sounds too early and the day is often full of traffic, chatter and senselessness, there is a globe of warmth within you that touches everything you touch.

After all this, the agony is over. Your life is far better and your weight problem is solved.

The Solution

Ask yourself these questions:

Cure 1:   Strong Nurturing
How do I feel? What do I need?   Do I need support?

Cure 2:   Effective Limits
Are my expectations reasonable?   Are my thoughts
positive and powerful? What is the essential pain?

Cure 3:   Body Pride
Am I avoiding weightist thoughts? Am I using words,
not my weight, to express myself?
Am I honoring and accepting my body?

Cure 4:   Good Health
How does my body feel? Am I taking care of my body?
Is my health care effective?

Cure 5:   Balanced Eating
Am I eating regularly? Am I eating only when hungry?
Is my food both healthy and pleasurable?

Cure 6:   Mastery Living
Am I physically active? Am I engaging in meaningful
activities? Am I taking time to restore myself?

The Solution

The Six Powerful Cures

MIND

Cure 1. Strong Nurturing
Effectiveness in getting your needs met.

3. Support   1. Feelings

2. Needs

Cure 2. Effective Limits
The strength to follow through.

3. Essential   1. Reasonable
   Pain   Expectations

2. Positive, Powerful Thoughts

BODY

Cure 3. Body Pride
Honoring and accepting your body.

3. Honor and   1. Avoid
   Accept   Weightism

2. Use Words, Not Weight

Cure 4. Good Health
Optimizing your physical vitality.

3. Health   1. Body
   Care   Awareness

2. Self-Care

LIFESTYLE

Cure 5. Balanced Eating
Eating for health and pleasure.

3. Health and   1. Regular
   Pleasure   Meals

2. Hunger

Cure 6. Mastery Living
An active and fulfilling lifestyle.

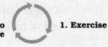

3. Time to   1. Exercise
   Restore

2. Meaningful Activities

Future Support

As you settle into using the six cures and approaching your weight in a very different way, you may want some additional support. You can share experiences with co-workers or friends who are using the method, but you may want more structure and guidance.

You can receive that guidance and a sense of community in mastering the method through participating in a Solution group. Teams of health professionals throughout the country conduct these programs after they have completed training and received certification in the method. Groups are conducted by registered dietitians to guide you through the lifestyle skills and social workers or psychologists to support you in mastering the mind and body skills.

The groups are full of warmth, humor and friendship. Confidentiality is honored and your physician provides medical approval. Solution groups meet for twelve weekly sessions of two hours each, usually in the early evening. Often participants are motivated to continue for two or more of these twelve-week programs because of the changes they see in their weight, health and happiness.

For centers near you offering Solution groups for adults, call The Institute for Health Solutions at 415-457-3331 or visit our Web site at www.weightsolution.com. For information on Shapedown programs for children or teens call 415-453-8886.

If there aren't yet any Solution groups in your community,

contact the chief clinical dietitians at the hospitals in your area and ask them about offering the program. Or contact the benefits department of your insurance carrier to ask for this service. In fact, you can have information sent to them about starting a program, just by calling our toll-free number.

Balanced Meals and Snacks

The most effective way for most people to move toward enhancing the health of their food is to use the Balanced Eating Food List on pages 291–292 as their menu. Turn there, if you will, and circle each food you enjoy. Then put them together in clusters that include at least one protein food (light protein or light milk food) per meal and enough fruits, vegetables and grains to satisfy you and support a gradual weight loss.

If you've been gaining weight, overeating or carrying your weight in the middle, when you are ready to lose weight, consider "shrinking your stomach" by selecting meals based on the menus that follow and having vegetables for snacks if you are hungry between meals. After a week of this way of eating, your insulin levels and gut peptide levels, which control appetite regulation, will have shifted, so your body won't demand as much food. It will then be far easier to accomplish weight loss.

After you sense that your appetite has diminished, you may decide to eat a little more or eat a few more heavier foods. You can do that safely and healthfully by asking yourself two questions:

"Do I really need to have it?"

"Is the essential pain of not having it too great for me?"

If the answers to these questions are yes, by all means make additions or substitutions that better meet your needs. If both a high-sugar and a high-fat food would please you equally, choose the high-sugar food.

If the answers to the two questions aren't both yes, then the meal you've already chosen is probably right for you at that time.

On the following pages there are menus and additional nutrition information. You probably don't need this information, but some of our participants enjoy it and want it, so I've included it in the book.

None of this information is meant to make you more anxious about your food. The orientation is not on restraining you from eating too much, but on being certain you receive *enough* of the nutrients you need for optimal health and happiness.

Balanced Breakfasts

2 slices whole wheat toast with ½ cup applesauce and cinnamon sugar

1 cup of 1% milk

coffee, decaf or tea

*   *   *

1 ounce whole grain cereal with 1 cup of 1% milk

orange juice

coffee, decaf or tea

*   *   *

1 bagel with no-fat cream cheese and blueberry jam

strawberries

coffee, decaf or tea

*   *   *

½ cup scrambled eggs (using egg substitute) and salsa

1 English muffin topped with blueberry jam

coffee, decaf or tea

*   *   *

1 carton raspberry nonfat yogurt (no sugar)

1 nonfat muffin

coffee, decaf or tea

*   *   *

two 4-inch pancakes topped with ½ cup strawberry yogurt (no sugar)

1 cup sliced strawberries

coffee, decaf or tea

½ cup hot cereal (oatmeal, whole wheat or farina)

½ cup 1% milk

½ cup apricot juice

coffee, decaf or tea

* * *

2 slices French toast: French bread, egg substitute and cinnamon

2 tablespoons low-sugar maple syrup

½ cup orange juice

* * *

breakfast shake: ½ cup 1% or nonfat milk, buttermilk or yogurt, 1 cup fresh fruit in any combination, 3 ice cubes, a dash of vanilla and sugar

1 slice whole wheat toast

coffee, decaf or tea

* * *

breakfast burrito: 1 corn tortilla, ½ cup nonfat refried beans, a few gratings of cheddar cheese and salsa

½ grapefruit

coffee, decaf or tea

* * *

½ cup cottage cheese (low-fat or nonfat)

½ cup fresh or canned pineapple

1 slice raisin bread

coffee, decaf or tea

* * *

1 cup fresh sliced fruit (any combination) topped with ½ cup flavored no-sugar yogurt and ¼ cup nonfat, juice-sweetened granola

coffee, decaf or tea

Balanced Lunches

large green salad with lots of vegetables and 3 ounces canned turkey, chicken or tuna nonfat dressing of your choice

1 slice whole wheat bread

nonfat milk

*   *   *

turkey sandwich on 2 slices rye, 7-grain or whole wheat bread

a large sweet orange or apple

diet soda

*   *   *

bean burrito: 1 tortilla, ½ cup nonfat refried beans, salsa, 1 ounce low-fat cheese

green salad with salsa

iced tea

*   *   *

nonfat potato chips

grilled chicken sandwich (barbecue or mustard sauce)

baby carrots

mineral water

*   *   *

1 cup leftover pasta salad: pasta, veggies, nonfat dressing

1 large chocolate graham cracker

mineral water

*   *   *

cream of vegetable soup made with any vegetables, chicken broth and evaporated low-fat milk

one 3-inch baguette

1 apple

iced tea

*   *   *

turkey salad with pieces of romaine lettuce, diced turkey, tomatoes and cucumbers

nonfat peppercorn or honey mustard dressing

whole wheat roll

diet soda

half of a turkey sandwich on 9-grain bread with lettuce and tomatoes

1 chocolate yogurt cone

coffee

*   *   *

1 latte made with nonfat milk and topped with chocolate powder

1 whole wheat bagel with low-fat sun-dried tomato cream cheese

1 banana

*   *   *

pita bread pocket stuffed with tempeh

fat-free tortilla chips

nonfat milk

1 peppermint candy

*   *   *

vegetarian chili or lentil soup

1 piece corn bread

1 large spinach and tomato salad with nonfat dressing

iced tea

*   *   *

instant pizza: pita bread topped with pizza sauce and low-fat mozzarella cheese

1 fresh pear

diet soda

Balanced Dinners

baked potato with chives, nonfat sour cream and pepper

barbecued ground sirloin, London broil or sirloin steak covered with mushrooms, onions and garlic sautéed in red wine

steamed broccoli with lemon and pepper

1 glass Merlot

1 cup nonfat tortilla chips

fish taco: large flour tortilla, 4 ounces fish, 1 ounce grated low-fat cheese, salsa

green salad with tomatoes, cilantro and cucumber

1 light beer

*   *   *

1 cup lentil soup

1 piece of corn bread with honey

1 cup nonfat milk

1 cup of strawberries with brown sugar and low-fat sour cream

water

*   *   *

1 cup pasta of your choice, marinara sauce and 4 ounces prawns or scallops

artichoke with nonfat mayonnaise

2 bread sticks

1 glass white wine

sliced cantaloupe and watermelon

*   *   *

1 large breast oven-fried chicken,

wild rice prepared without oil

fruit salad: bananas, apples, pears, cherries and oranges

green salad with nonfat dressing

2 chocolate kisses

hot tea

*   *   *

popcorn (air-popped) and mineral water

4 ounces barbecued salmon

potato salad made with potatoes, onions, celery, nonfat mayonnaise and spices

2 slices French bread

coffee

1 fresh pear with crumbled blue cheese

1 baked potato stuffed with ½ cup low-fat or nonfat ricotta cheese

broccoli and salsa

1 large fruit salad

2 bread sticks

water

*   *   *

1 cup black beans, Haitian style

½ cup brown rice

fresh mango, bananas and strawberries

2 gingersnaps

lemon-flavored mineral water

*   *   *

1 cup spinach-and-cheese-stuffed tortellini

½ cup marinara sauce

fresh asparagus with lemon

1 slice French bread

coffee

2 chocolate graham crackers

*   *   *

barbecued chicken drumstick and breast

corn on the cob (no butter)

spinach salad with orange slices

decaf

angel food cake

*   *   *

pork tenderloin with Chinese sweet-and-sour sauce

½ cup white rice

mixed grilled vegetables: mushrooms, red potatoes, carrots and zucchini

raspberries topped with low-fat flavored yogurt

tea

Balanced Snacks

1 cup of red and green seedless grapes

tender-crisp asparagus, chilled and dipped in lemon yogurt

celery stuffed with nonfat cream cheese and topped with garlic powder or paprika

little red potatoes microwaved and chilled, sliced in half and sprinkled with lemon

sliced cantaloupe and kiwi

peppers and onions, sautéed, and a mashed handful of cherries

pineapple spears

iced vegetable or tomato juice with a celery stalk stirrer

a wedge of lettuce dipped in a favorite nonfat dressing

an artichoke with nonfat mayonnaise

1 100 percent fruit juice bar

crisp long green beans, cold, dipped in warm marinara sauce

a large bowl of strawberries

1 microwaved ear of corn, steaming hot

Balanced Meals and Snacks

Meals

1. One or more servings of foods that are high in protein (light proteins or light milk foods).

2. The amount of grains, fruits and vegetables in order to:

- meet your daily nutritional needs (5-5-2-2).

- feel satisfied, not full when you stop eating.

- lose an average of one pound per week.

3. Add heavier foods if you *need* more food pleasure and the *essential pain* of not having them is too difficult.

Snacks

1. Foods with a low emotional payoff: fruits and vegetables.

2. The amount of these foods that:

- keeps your energy high between meals.

- allows your hunger to return by the next meal.

One Serving Equals . . .

The serving sizes listed below are used to ensure you get <u>enough</u> nutrition. They are *not* used to <u>limit</u> how much you eat.

Fruits and Vegetables
- 1 piece (e.g., one banana, one carrot)
- ½ cup vegetables or fruit juice
- ¼ cup dried fruit
- 1 cup of leafy raw vegetables

Grains
- 1 slice of bread, ½ bagel, 1 small roll
- ½ cup hot cereal, 1 ounce ready-to-eat cereal
- ½ cup pasta or rice, 4 crackers, 1 small tortilla

Proteins
- 3 ounces fish, light meats, turkey or chicken breast
- ½ cup beans, 1 cup bean soup
- 1 veggie burger, 1 slice tofu, ½ cup egg substitute

Milk Foods
- 1 cup milk or yogurt
- ½ cup cottage cheese or ricotta cheese
- 1 ounce cheese, ¼ cup nonfat cream cheese

Health Enhancers

Light foods that contain phytochemicals

beta carotene
yellow foods: carrots, winter squash, sweet
potatoes, apricots, papaya, cantaloupe, mango
dark green foods: broccoli, Brussels sprouts,
spinach, dark leafy greens

Vitamin C
oranges, tangerines, grapefruit, kiwi, raspberries,
blackberries, pineapple, broccoli, tomatoes, peppers

fiber
whole wheat bread and cereal, bran cereals, wheat
bran, oatmeal, beans, lentils, dried peas, apples,
strawberries, blackberries, raspberries

cruciferous vegetables
broccoli, Brussels sprouts, bok choy, cabbage, kale,
cauliflower, radishes, mustard greens

omega-3 fatty acids
(linolenic acid, EPA and DHA)
fish *contains all three of these omega-3 fatty acids;
small amounts of one of these fatty acids, linolenic,
are in:* vegetables, beans, pork, veal, low-fat cheese,
wheat germ, oats, corn

other health enhancers
(phytosterols, lycopene, isoflavones, allylic sulfides)
garlic, onions, ginger, leeks, chives, watermelon, red
peppers, tomatoes, pink grapefruit, soybeans, tofu,
soy milk, tempeh

Pleasure Enhancers

Light foods that bring pleasure

Pour on the sweetness
a teaspoon of sugar, jam, honey, cinnamon sugar, brown
sugar, molasses, vanilla

Add a touch of fat
less than a teaspoon of butter, oil, mayonnaise, salad dressing,
nut butters, a few gratings of cheese

Add some richness without fat
nonfat cream cheese, nonfat mayonnaise, nonfat bean dips,
fruit spreads, nonfat dips, nonfat sour cream

Light comfort foods
nonfat frozen yogurt, nonfat ice cream, Popsicles, fruit ices,
sorbet, sugar-free Jell-O, sugar-free pudding

Satisfying the munchies
nonfat potato chips and nonfat onion dip,
nonfat corn chips and salsa or bean dip,
platter of raw veggies and nonfat garlic or mustard dip

Making food savory
garlic, onions, horseradish, Worchestershire sauce, salsa,
pepper sauce, mustard, daikon, ginger, turnips, fresh and
dried herbs and spices

Tried and true flavor boosters
pepper, lemon, lime, vinegars, soy sauce, barbecue sauce,
ketchup, sugar plus vinegar, honey plus lemon, salt (if you are
not salt sensitive)

Wine and spirits
up to 1 drink per day for women and up to 2 for men. A drink
is 4 oz. wine, 12 oz. light beer, or 1 oz. liquor

Wet refreshers
mineral water, fruit spritzers, soda water, diet soda, ice tea, hot
tea, coffee, decaffeinated coffee, espresso drinks with nonfat
milk, and at least 6 cups of water per day

Research

Several studies were conducted at the University of California, San Francisco, in the course of developing this work. One study evaluated the effects of the Shapedown program, which is the child and adolescent version of the method. The study followed 64 teens and their families for a year after a fourteen-week program. Depression, diet and exercise patterns and self-esteem all improved. After the program, the weight of adolescents continued to decrease even a year later.

Another study evaluated a broad range of characteristics of obese adolescents participating in the program and found that other than genetics, what contributed most to their weight was not diet, exercise or depression but the connection they made with themselves and others.

The research of greatest relevance to this book is the two-year follow-up study of the first groups of men and women who were treated with *The Solution* at the university. When we compared the effectiveness of diet and exercise programs to *The Solution*, *The Solution* appeared to produce longer lasting results.

With any of the methods studied, weight decreased during treatment, which is what most weight-loss studies reveal. When people receive support for eating healthfully and exercising regularly, they usually shed some weight, only to regain it within a year or two. As such, the effectiveness of any weight treatment is based on the changes that are sustained *after* the warmth of the group fades, *after* the external limits of prepared foods vanish and

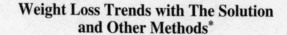

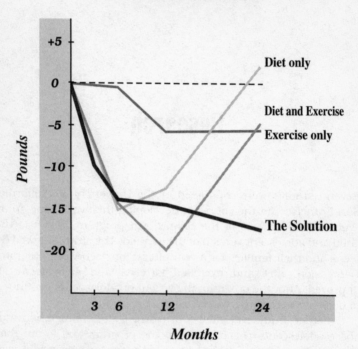

Weight Loss Trends with The Solution and Other Methods*

* Weight changes for treatment groups at 3, 12 and 24 months adapted from Skender, M.L. et al., *Journal of the American Dietetic Association* 1996;96:342–346, and Mellin, L. M., Dickey, L. and Croughan-Minihane, M.M., *Journal of the American Dietetic Association* 1996; 96:A-31.

after the personal trainer takes a hike. In this case Solution group participants continued to lose weight, while those in traditional diet and exercise programs regained most or all the weight they had lost.

There were immediate benefits to these participants in health and happiness, but what is of importance is the results that were seen two years later. Not only had most of the participants expe-

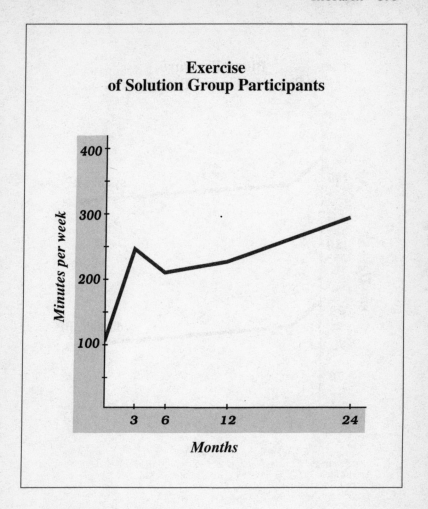

**Exercise
of Solution Group Participants**

rienced weight loss that had lasted, but most reported a broad
spectrum of positive life changes.

What was impressive was not just the objective data, but the
quality of the responses. Their progress seemed not hard won,
but the natural result of changes within. What's more, those
who mastered the cures during the sessions were the ones who
two years later had the greatest magnitude of weight change and
the most consistent patterns of broad-spectrum change in their
lives.

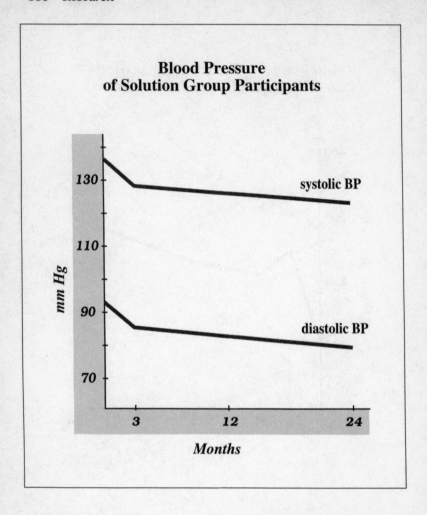

**Blood Pressure
of Solution Group Participants**

This testing followed 29 people and included data on 22 of those who completed the training. Surely longer-term studies with matched control groups are in order to fully evaluate the effectiveness of the method. In fact, John Foreyt, Ph.D., and Ken Goodrick, Ph.D., obesity researchers at Baylor Medical College in Houston, Texas, are collaborating with the University of California, San Francisco School of Medicine, to seek funding to study the method further.

Immediate Changes with *The Solution*

(Changes Reported After 12 Weeks)

Lost Weight   91 percent lost weight right away, averaging a 10-pound weight loss.

Felt Happier   levels of depression decreased 63 percent (Beck Depression Inventory).

Improved
Health   blood pressure dropped an average of 7 mm Hg and became normal in one-third of those whose blood pressure had been high.

Exercised
More   95 percent exercised more; on the average they increased their exercise more than two hours per week.

Longer-Term Changes with
The Solution
(Changes Reported Two Years Later)

Better Health

Maintained a Weight Loss	77%
Improved Health and Vitality	77%
Decreased Blood Pressure[1]	67%
Exercise More[2]	68%

Greater Happiness

Felt Happier	91%
Improved Relationships	86%
Coped Better with Work	86%
Deepened Spirituality	73%

More Success

More Productive at Work	54%
Spent More Responsibly	59%
Began Saving More	41%
Used Substances Less[3]	63%

1. *Both* systolic and diastolic blood pressures decreased 5 mm Hg or more. On the average blood pressure decreased 13.75 mm Hg (systolic) and 14.5 mm Hg (diastolic).

2. Increased an average of more than three hours of exercise per week.

3. Percent of those who smoked, drank heavily or used drugs who reported stopping or significantly improving their substance use.

Selected Readings

Too much reading on topics related to the method may not be in your best interests. At times learning more and gaining more insight is comforting, but the energy you expend in these intellectual pursuits can actually divert attention from the far more difficult and far more powerful task of changing—that is, mastering the cures.

With that said, I've collected a few references to exceptional books you may enjoy. I've suggested several that may help deepen your understanding of some of the underlying principles of the cures. In addition, I've suggested some excellent books on healthy, pleasurable eating and safe, effective physical activity as well as several other good sources of information.

Cure 1: Strong Nutrition

Gray, John. *What You Feel, You Can Heal: A Guide for Enriching Relationships.* Mill Valley, CA: Heart Publishing, 1994. This is a picture book that uses humor and straight talk to get right to the heart of the issue of nurturing. Men, in particular, enjoy this book because of its humor. A must-read!

Meadow, Rosalyn, and Weiss, Lillie. *Women's Conflicts About Eating and Sexuality.* New York: Haworth Press, 1992. Although this book goes awry when it dabbles in weight management, its description of issues of sexuality and eating is enlightening. A good read if you are a woman who is not currently sexually fulfilled.

Miller, Alice. *The Drama of the Gifted Child: The Search for the True Self.* New York: Basic Books, 1990. This classic book examines how narcissistic, self-absorbed parents affect their children's development, particularly in the areas of nurturing and limits.

Cure 2: Effective Limits

Gray, John. *Men Are from Mars, Women Are from Venus: A Practical Guide for Improving Communication and Getting What You Want in Your Relationships.* New York: HarperCollins Publishers, 1992. Just the way you lovingly embrace the part of you that is still demanding, needy, self-pitying or hostile, this book points out the empathy and compassion we must muster, and the essential pain we must face, to reap fulfillment in our relationships.

McCann, Eileen, and Shannon, Douglas. *The Two-Step: The Dance Toward Intimacy.* New York: Grove Press, 1985. If you think your relationships become power struggles, this book will knock your socks off. It's composed mainly of drawings, and the drawings are worth millions of words. The book powerfully depicts the funny and not-so-funny patterns and struggles in which we find ourselves. This book is a jewel.

Stuart, Richard, and Jacobson, Barbara. *Weight, Sex and Marriage: A Delicate Balance.* New York: Simon & Schuster, 1989. This classic book discusses the issues of control and boundaries in a marriage that keep one partner heavy. Although the solutions provided are dated, the description of the dynamics is right on target.

Cure 3: Body Pride

Erdman, Cheri. *Nothing to Lose: A Guide to Sane Living in a Larger Body.* San Francisco: HarperSanFrancisco, 1995. Support for the practical aspects of body pride before you reclaim your biological body size.

Freedman, Rita. *Bodylove: Learning to Like Our Looks—and Ourselves.* New York: Harper & Row, 1989. This straightforward book on accepting and honoring our bodies provides some interesting information about this important issue.

Wolf, Naomi. *The Beauty Myth: How Images of Beauty Are Used Against Women.* New York: Anchor Books, 1991. This is the story of the evolution of lookism and the changes in expectations for women's shape and size.

Cure 4: Good Health

Ornish, Dean. *Dr. Dean Ornish's Program for Reversing Heart Disease*. New York: Ballantine Books, 1990. This revolutionary program for reversing heart disease has become the state-of-the art treatment for heart disease. For a listing of clinical programs in your area, write to The Preventive Medicine Research Institute, 600 Bridgeway, Sausalito, CA 94960.

U.S. Department of Agriculture. *Report of the Dietary Guidelines Advisory Committee on the Dietary Guidelines for Americans*, 1995. Single copies may be obtained at no cost from Debbie Reed, National Program Staff, BARC-West, Building 005, Room 215, Beltsville, MD 20705 or purchased from the National Technical Information Service, 5285 Port Royal Road, Springfield, VA 22161, phone: 1-703-487-4650. This report, issued every five years, is the U.S. government's statement of what we should eat and why.

Cure 5: Balanced Eating

Cooking Light Cookbooks: Microwave, Poultry, and Salads and Dressings. New York: Warner Books, 1991. These cookbooks are inexpensive paperbacks that reflect the same good-tasting low-fat fare presented in the monthly magazine *Cooking Light*.

Goor, Ron. *Eater's Choice*. Boston: Houghton Mifflin, 1992. This book is actually an approach to heart disease prevention, but half of it is devoted to low-fat recipes that have received positive reviews.

Niethimmer, Carolyn. *Great Taste: Healthy Cooking from Canyon Ranch*. Tucson, AZ: Canyon Ranch Enterprises, 1995. These recipes are very low in fat, and the food is both delicious to eat and pleasing to behold. Create an elegant spa of your own at home.

Ornish, Dean. *Everyday Cooking with Dr. Dean Ornish*. New York: HarperCollins, 1996. In previous books, you've seen Dr. Ornish's recipes from the San Francisco Bay Area's most avant-garde cooks who whip up melt-in-your-mouth nonfat vegetarian fare. This new cookbook has all the flavor and none of the fuss. Quick, easy and delicious recipes you can re-create yourself.

Cure 6: Mastery Living

Bailey, Covert. *Smart Exercise: Burning Fat, Getting Fit.* Boston: Houghton Mifflin, 1994. Covert Bailey gives no-nonsense answers to commonly asked exercise questions. It's an informative, easy-to-read book.

Heler, Stuart, and Surrenda, David Sheppard. *Retooling on the Run: Real Change for Leaders with No Time.* Berkeley: Frog, Ltd., 1994. Outlines a new foundation for leadership that begins with personal change. Includes a whole range of body pride and body empowerment exercises.

Leonard, George. *Mastery: The Keys to Success and Long-Term Fulfillment.* New York: Penguin Books, 1992. This remarkable book draws on Zen philosophy to portray a way of living that leads to excellence.

Louden, Jennifer. *The Woman's Comfort Book: A Self-Nurturing Guide for Restoring Balance in Your Life.* New York: HarperCollins, 1992. Men too will enjoy this fun, idea-filled work, which provides every imaginable way to nurture yourself.

Peck, M. Scott. *The Road Less Traveled: A New Psychology of Love, Traditional Values and Spiritual Growth.* New York: Simon & Schuster, 1978. If you have not yet discovered this classic book, it is a must-read.

Additional sources of information

The Weight-Control Information Network (WIN) is a service of the National Institute of Diabetes and Digestive and Kidney Diseases (NIDDK), part of the National Institutes of Health. Authorized by Congress, WIN assembles and disseminates information on weight control, obesity and nutritional disorders. Write to WIN, 1 WIN WAY, Bethesda, MD 20892-4665, or call 1-301-570-2177 to speak with an information specialist. To receive automated information, including up-to-date messages on obesity research and free copies of publications, call 1-800-946-8098, fax 1-301-570-2186 or send e-mail to WINNIDDK @ aol.com.

The National Heart, Lung and Blood Institute Information Center is another NIH service that provides free information about nutrition, activity and overweight. Phone: 1-301-251-1222. Fax: 1-301-251-1223.

The American Dietetic Association offers a hotline through which you can speak to registered dietitians about nutrition and diet or receive information and referrals. The number is 1-800-366-1655.

The Council on Size and Weight Discrimination publishes resource directories and bibliographies on eating disorders and weightism. Write to them at P.O. Box 305, Mount Marion, NY 12456 or call 1-914-679-1209 or fax 1-914-679-1206.

The National Association of Anorexia and Associated Disorders operates a hotline for information about eating disorders, including referrals to treatment and support groups. Write to them at P.O. Box 7, Highland Park, IL 60035 or call 1-708-831-3438 or fax 1-708-433-4632.

Bibliography

Astrup, A., and Raben, A. 1995. Carbohydrate and obesity. *International Journal of Obesity* 19, Suppl 5:S27-S37.

Atkinson, R. L., and Hubbard, V. S. 1994. Report on the NIH workshop on pharmacologic treatment of obesity. *American Journal of Clinical Nutrition* 60:53-156.

Blair, S. N. 1989. Physical fitness and all cost mortality: a prospective study of healthy men and women. *Journal of the American Medical Association* 262:2395–2401.

Bolton-Smith, C., and Woodward, M. 1994. Dietary composition and fat to sugar ratios in relation to obesity. *International Journal of Obesity* 18:820–828.

Bouchard, C., Tremblay, A., Despres, J. P., Nadeau, A., Lupien, P., Theriault, G., Dussault, J., Moorjani, S., Pinault, S., and Fournier, G. 1990. The response to long-term overfeeding in identical twins. *New England Journal of Medicine* 322:1477–1482.

Brownell, K. D., Kelman, J. H., and Stunkard, A. J. 1983. Treatment of obese children with and without their mothers: changes in weight and blood pressure. *Pediatrics* 7, 1:515–523.

Bruch, H. 1973. *Eating Disorders: Obesity, Anorexia Nervosa and the Person Within.* New York: Basic Books.

———. 1957. *The Importance of Overweight.* New York: W.W. Norton.

Bruch, H., and Touraine, G. 1940. Obesity in childhood: V. The family frame of obese children. *Psychosomatic Medicine* 11:142–206.

Calam, R. M., and Slade, P. D. 1989. Sexual experience and eating problems in female undergraduates. *International Journal of Eating Disorders* 8:391–397.

Carey, W. B., Hegvik, R. L., and McDevitt, S. C. 1988. Temperamental factors associated with rapid weight gain and obesity in middle school children. *Developmental and Behavioral Pediatrics* 9:194–198.

Ching, P. L., Willett, W. C., Rimm, E. B., Colditz, G. N., Gortmaker, S. L., and Stampfor, M. J. 1996. Activity level and risk of overweight in male health professionals. *American Journal of Public Health* 86:25–30.

Christoffel, K. K., and Forsyth, B. W. C. 1989. Mirror image of environmental deprivation: severe childhood obesity of psychosocial origin. *Child Abuse & Neglect* 13:249–256.

Dietz, W. H., Jr., and Gortmaker, S. L. 1985. Do we fatten our children at the television set? Obesity and television viewing in children and adolescents. *Pediatrics* 75:807–812.

Drenowski, A., Brunzell, J. D., Sande, K., Iverius, R. M., and Greenwood, M. R. C. 1985. Sweet tooth reconsidered: taste preferences in human obesity. *Physiological Behavior* 35:617–622.

Drug Facts and Comparisons. 1996. St. Louis: Facts and Comparisons.

Epstein, L. H., Klein, K. R., and Wisniewski, L. 1994. Child and parent factors that influence psychological problems of obese children. *International Journal of Eating Disorders* 15:151–158.

Epstein, L. H., Valoski, A., Wing, R. R., and McCurley, J. 1990. Ten-year follow-up of behavioral, family-based treatment for obese children. *Journal of the American Medical Association* 264:2519–2523.

Epstein, L. H., Wing, R. R., Koeske, R., and Valoski, A. 1987. Long-term effects of family-based treatment of childhood obesity. *Journal of Consulting and Clinical Psychology* 55:91–95.

Ewbank, P. P., Darga, L. L., and Lucas, C. P. 1995. Physical activity as a predictor of weight maintenance in previously obese subjects. *Obesity Research* 3:257–263.

Felitti, V. J. 1993. Childhood sexual abuse, depression and family dysfunction in adult obese patients: a case controlled study. *Southern Medical Journal* 86:732–736.

———. 1991. Long-term medical consequences of incest, rape and molestation. *Southern Medical Journal* 84:328–331.

Flodmark, C. E., Ohlsson, T., Ryden, O., and Sveger, T. 1993. Prevention of progression to severe obesity in a group of obese school children treated with family therapy. *Pediatrics* 9, 1:880–884.

Froideavaux, F., Schutz, Y., Christin, L., and Jequier, E. 1993. Energy expenditure in obese females before weight loss, after refeeding and in the weight relapse period. *American Journal of Clinical Nutrition* 57:35–42.

Garn, S. M. 1985. Continuities and changes in fatness from infancy through adulthood. *Current Problems in Pediatrics* 15:1–47.

Garn, S. M., and Clark, D. C. 1976. Trends in fatness and origins of obesity. *Pediatrics* 57:443–456.

Gortmaker, S. L., Dietz, W. H., Jr., and Cheung, L. W. 1990. Inactivity, diet and the fattening of America. *Journal of the American Dietetic Association* 97:1247–1252.

Guy-Grand, B., Apfelbaum, M., Crepaldo, G., Gries, A., Lefebvre, P., and Turner, P. 1989. International trial of long-term dexfenfluramine in obesity. *The Lancet* 11:8672:1142–1144.

Jenkins, D. J. A., Wolever, T. M. S., Buckley, G., Lam, K. Y., Giudici, S., Kalmusky, J., Jenkins, A. L., Patten, R. L., Bird, J., Wong, G. S., and Josse, G. 1988. Low-glycemic-index starch foods in the diabetic diet. *American Journal of Clinical Nutrition* 48:248–254.

Kernberg, O. F. 1970. Factors in the psychoanalytic treatment of narcissistic personalities. *Journal of the American Psychoanalytic Association* 18:51–85.

Kesten, D., and Armstrong, L. The protective power of plants. *Veggie Life's Nourish,* October/November 1995.

Kinston, W., Loader, P., Miller, L., and Rein, L. 1988. Interaction in families with obese children. *Journal of Psychosomatic Research* 4/5:513–532.

Kinston, W., Miller, L., Loarder, P., and Wolff, O. 1990. Evaluating sex differences in childhood obesity by using a family systems approach. *Family Systems Medicine* 4:371–386.

Klesges, R. C., Shelton, M. L., Klesges, L. M. 1993. Effects of television on metabolic rate: potential implications for childhood obesity. *Pediatrics* 9, 1:281–286.

Kuczmarski, R. J., Flegal, K. M., Campbell, S. M., Johnson, C. L. 1994. Increasing prevalence of overweight among U.S. adults. The National Health and Nutrition Examination Survey, 1960 to 1991. *Journal of the American Medical Association* 272:205–211.

Lipschitz, D. A., ed. 1995. *Clinics in Geriatric Medicine. Nutrition, Aging, and Age-Dependent Diseases.* 11, 4. Philadephia: W.B. Saunders.

Lissau, I., Breum, L., and Sorensen, T. I. A. 1993. Maternal attitude to sweet eating habits and risk of overweight in offspring: a ten-year prospective population study. *International Journal of Obesity* 17:125–129.

Mahler, M. 1968. *On Human Symbiosis and the Vicissitudes of Individuation.* New York: International Universities Press.

Mahler, M. S., Pine, F., and Bergman, A. 1975. *The Psychological Birth of the Human Infant: Symbiosis and Individuation.* New York: Basic Books.

Masoro, E. J., ed. 1995. *Handbook of Physiology: A Critical, Comprehensive Presentation of Physiological Knowledge and Concepts. Section 11: Aging.* New York: American Physiological Society, Oxford University Press.

Melbin, T., and Vuille, J. C. 1989. Further evidence of an association between psychosocial problems and increase in relative weight between 7 and 10 years. *Acta Paediatrica Scandinavica* 78:576–580.

———. 1989. Rapidly developing overweight in school children as an indicator of psychosocial stress. *Acta Paediatrica Scandinavica* 78:568–575.

Mellin, L. 1993. To: President Clinton Re: Combating Childhood Obesity. *Journal of the American Dietetic Association* 93:265–266.

Mellin, L. M., and Frost, L. 1992. Child and adolescent obesity: the nurse practitioner's use of the Shapedown method. *Journal of Pediatric Health Care* 6:187–193.

Mellin, L., Dickey L., and Croughan-Minihane, S. 1996. Cognitive-emotive training: developmental testing of the Shapedown method for adults. *Journal of the American Dietetic Association* 96:A–31.

Mellin, L. M., Slinkard, L. A., and Irwin, C. E. 1987. Adolescent obesity intervention: validation of the Shapedown program. *Journal of the American Dietetic Association* 87:333–337.

Miller, A. 1979. Depression and grandiosity as related forms of narcissistic disturbances. *International Review of Psychoanalysis* 6:1–76.

Miller, Alice. 1990. *The Drama of the Gifted Child: The Search for the True Self.* New York: Basic Books.

Minuchin, S. 1978. *Psychosomatic Families: Anorexia Nervosa in Context.* Cambridge: Harvard University Press.

Minuchin, S., Baker, L., Rosman, B. L., Liebman, R., Milman, L., and Todd, T. C. 1975. A conceptual model of psychosomatic illness in children. *Archives of General Psychiatry* 32:1031–1038.

Paffenbarger, R. F., Jr. 1986. Physical activity, all-cause mortality, and longevity of college alumni. *New England Journal of Medicine* 3, 14:605–613.

Raben, A., and Astrup A. 1995. Impact of 14 day ad libitum sucrose-rich, fat-rich or recommended diet on energy intake and body composition in post-obese and controls. *International Journal of Obesity* 19, Suppl. 2:33.

Richards, M. H., Casper, R. C., and Larson, R. 1990. Weight and eating concerns among pre- and young adolescent boys and girls. *Journal of Adolescent Health Care* 11:203–209.

Roe, Daphne A., M.D. 1994. *Handbook of Drug and Nutrient Interactions: A Reference and Study Guide.* Chicago: American Dietetic Association.

Satir, V. 1983. *Conjoint Family Therapy.* Palo Alto: Science and Behavior Books.

Shargel, L. 1993. *Comprehensive Pharmacy Review,* 2d ed, Philadelphia: Harwal Publishing.

Skender, M. L., Goodrick, G. K., Del Juncom, D. J., Reeves, R. S., Darnell, L., Gotto, A. N., Jr., and Foreyt, J. P. 1996. Comparison of 2-year weight loss trends in behavioral treatment of obesity: diet, exercise, and combination interventions. *Journal of the American Dietetic Association* 96:342–346.

Sorensen, T. I. A., Holst, C., Stunkard, A. J., and Skovgaard, L. T. 1992. Correlation of body mass index of adult adoptees and their biological and adoptive relatives. *International Journal of Obesity and Related Metabolic Disorders* 16:227–236.

Spritz, A., Heymesfield, S., and Blank, R. 1995. Drug therapy for obesity: clinical considerations. *Endocrine Practice* 1:274–278.

Stunkard, A. J., Marris, J. R., Pedersen, N. L., and McClearn, G. E. 1990. A separated twin study of the body mass index. *New England Journal of Medicine* 322:1483–1487.

Tappy, L., and Jequier, E. 1992. The components of energy expenditure in human obesity. *Acta Clinica Belgia.* Suppl. 14:13–17.

Volger, G. P., Sorensen, T. A., Stunkard, A. J., Srinivasan, M. R., Rao, D. L. 1995. Influences of genes and shared family environment on adult body mass index assessed in an adoption study by a comprehensive path model. *International Journal of Obesity and Related Metabolic Disorders* 19:40–45.

Zelasko, C. J. 1995. Exercise for weight loss: what are the facts? *Journal of the American Dietetic Association* 95:1414–1417.

Index

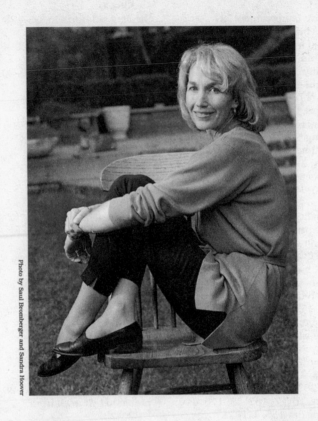

LAUREL MELLIN, M.A., R.D., is an associate clinical professor of family and community medicine and pediatrics at the University of California, San Francisco School of Medicine where she developed *The Solution*. She lives in Marin County, CA.